ANTI- INFLAMMATORY
DIET COOKBOOK

Easy Recipes to Fight Inflammation with a 30-day meal plan

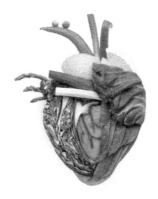

Marta Harter

Table of Contents

Introduction

This book offers tried-and-true instructions and ideas for preparing and serving breakfast, lunch, and supper to those on an anti-inflammatory diet. People with significant conditions such as rheumatoid arthritis are returned to an anti-inflammatory diet.

Many deadly diseases, including Alzheimer's, cancer, rheumatoid arthritis, and cardiovascular disease, are caused by chronic inflammation in the human body. Inflammation is a natural reaction to a foreign invader or wounded tissue. Inflammation causes swelling, redness, and pain. However, when it lasts for a lengthy period of time or appears for no apparent reason, the body suffers. Chronic inflammation may be caused by a variety of unhealthy lifestyle choices, including smoking, working long hours, not getting enough exercise, and eating badly.

A patient must stick to an anti-inflammatory diet to fight inflammation and keep it from getting worse. Aside from helping people lose weight, the diet plan can also help keep people from getting sick. It helps keep the health of a patient in check.

An anti-inflammatory diet should include between 2,000 and 3,000 calories, 67 grams of fat, and 2,300 milligrams of salt per day. These calories should come from 50% carbohydrates, 20% protein, and 30% fat. Good sources of carbohydrates include whole-wheat grains, sweet potatoes, squash, bulgur wheat, beans, and brown rice.

The majority of your fat intake should come from fish and dishes prepared with extra-virgin olive oil or organic canola oil. Soybeans and other soy-based entire products include protein.

This diet eliminates all forms of fast food and processed foods. This prohibition also applies to pork, beef, butter, cream, and margarine.

Additionally, the anti-inflammatory diet should have less processed sugar for diabetics and reduced cholesterol (however Omega-3, which is present in a variety of fish, is a beneficial cholesterol) for those with heart conditions.

One of the advantages of an anti-inflammatory diet is that it incorporates fresh foods rich in phytonutrients, which help to avoid degenerative diseases. The inclusion of Omega-3 fatty acids in the diet plan also produces cardiovascular benefits. These fatty acids help to avoid cardiac problems and lower levels of "bad" cholesterol and blood pressure.

The anti-inflammatory diet is good for diabetics, which is an additional benefit. This diet is great for diabetics since it avoids processed sugar and sugary foods. Although the diet does not dramatically decrease weight, it reduces the patient's likelihood of becoming obese. This is due to the inclusion of natural fruits and vegetables and the restriction of meat and other processed meals.

30-Day Meal Plan

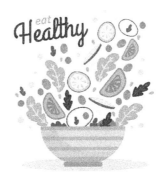

DAY 1

BREAKFAST

Vanilla Turmeric Orange Juice

Prep/Cook Time:5 mins, Servings: 2

Ingredients

- 3 oranges, peeled + q uartered
- 1 cup unsweetened almond milk
- 1 t vanilla extract
- 1/2 t cinnamon
- 1/4 t turmeric
- Pinch of pepper

Instructions

1. Place all the ingredients in a blender.
2. Blend until smooth, then pour into a glass and serve.

Nutrition Info

Calories: 156, Cholesterol: 65mg, Carbohydrate: 8.42g, Protein: 7.37

LUNCH

Smashed Chickpea Avocado Salad Sandwich with Cranberries + Lemon

Prep/Cook Time: 5 mins, Servings: 2

Ingredients

- 1 – 15 oz can chickpeas, rinsed and drained
- 1 large ripe avocado
- 2 teaspoon freshly squeezed lemon juice

- 1/4 cup dried cranberries
- Freshly ground salt & pepper, to taste

OPTIONAL:

- 4 slices of your favorite whole grain bread (or gluten free)

Toppings:

- Arugula, red onion, or spinach

Instructions

1   In a medium bowl, smash chickpeas with a fork. Add in avocado and use fork to smash again until avocado is smooth, yet still contains a few chunky pieces. Stir in lemon juice and cranberries. Season with salt and pepper to taste. Place in refrigerator until ready to serve (best within 1-2 days).

2   When ready to serve, toast bread then spread 1/2 chickpea avocado salad over 1 slice. Top with arugula, red onion or spinach, if desired. Add other toasted slice on top, then cut in half and enjoy!

Nutrition Info

Calories: 406, Fat: 15.3g, Carbohydrates: 60.5g, Sugar: 10.7g, Fiber: 17.3g, Protein: 12.3g

----

DINNER

Baked Buffalo cauliflower recipe

Prep/Cook Time: 50 mins, Servings 2-4

Ingredients

- 1 medium cauliflower, cut into bite-size pieces (approximately 4 cups)
- 1/4 cup banana flour

- 1/4 cup water
- Pinch of salt and pepper
- 2 tablespoons butter, melted
- 1/2 cup hot sauce

For serving (optional):

- blue cheese or ranch dressing

Instructions

1. Preheat the oven to 425 degrees.
2. Whisk the flour, water, salt, and pepper together in a large mixing bowl.
3. Add the cauliflower to the flour and water mixture and toss to coat. Place on a foil-lined baking sheet, and bake flipping once, for approximately 15 minutes.
4. Meanwhile, mix the butter and hot sauce together in a small bowl. Drizzle the sauce over the baked cauliflower. Return to the oven and bake for an additional 20 minutes. Serve warm with your favorite dressing on the side, if desired.

Nutrition Info

Calories 369, Carbohydrates 17g, Fiber 10g, Sugar 2g, Protein 11g

DAY 2

BREAKFAST

No-Bake Turmeric Protein Donuts

Prep/Cook Time: 50 mins, Servings: 8 mini donuts

Ingredients

- 1 1/2 cups raw cashews
- 1/2 cup (7 pieces) Medjool dates, pitted
- 1 T vanilla protein powder
- 1/4 cup shredded coconut
- 2 t maple syrup
- 1/4 t vanilla essence
- 1 t turmeric powder
- 1/4 cup dark chocolate (for topping)

Instructions

1. Combine all ingredients (except the chocolate) in a food processor and process on high until a smooth and sticky cookie dough forms.
2. Roll batter into eight balls and firmly press into silicone donut mold. Cover mold with plastic wrap and place in freezer 30 minutes to set.
3. For the chocolate topping, pour a cup of water into a saucepan and bring to a boil.
4. Then place a smaller saucepan on top of the pan and add the chocolate to the bowl. Stir gently until the chocolate is completely melted.
5. Once set, remove donuts from mold, drizzle with dark chocolate and store in an airtight container in the fridge.

Nutrition Info

Calories 342, Fat 19g, Saturated Fat 5g, Carbohydrates 7g, Fiber 1g,

Sugar 1g, Protein 31g

LUNCH

Turmeric Chai Chia Pudding

Prep Time: 3 minutes, Servings: 2-4 servings

Ingredients

- 1.5 cups cashew milk or other nut milk
- 1/3 cup chia seeds
- 2 tbsp maple syrup
- 1 tsp ground turmeric
- 1/2 tsp cinnamon
- 1/8 tsp ground cardamom
- 1/8 tsp ground cloves

Instructions

1 Mix all the ingredients together in a bowl. Pour in to individual bowls or jars.
2 Let set overnight.
3 Eat plain or top with fruit and nuts.

Nutrition Info

Calories 164, Carbohydrates 13g, Fiber 2g, Sugar 1g, Protein 13g

----

DINNER

Korean Grilled Mackere

Prep/Cook Time 1 h, 4 servings

Ingredients

- 2 tablespoons Korean chile paste

- 1 tablespoon canola oil
- 1 tablespoon reduced-sodium soy sauce
- 2 teaspoons rice vinegar
- 1 teaspoon grated fresh ginger
- 2 whole mackerel (about 1½ pounds each) or 4 whole rainbow trout (about 5 ounces each), cleaned and butterflied, tails left on

Instructions

1   Whisk chile paste, oil, soy sauce, vinegar and ginger in a small bowl until smooth. Transfer 2 tablespoons marinade to a small bowl and set aside. Open each fish like a book, exposing the flesh. Place in a large pan or on a baking sheet and spread the remaining marinade over the flesh. Marinate in the refrigerator for 30 minutes to 1 hour. About 20 minutes before you're ready to grill, preheat grill to high or prepare a charcoal fire. Brush the grill rack clean and oil it well. Grill the fish, flesh-side down, for 3 minutes. Flip with a large spatula, spread the reserved marinade over the fish and grill until opaque in the center, 3 to 4 minutes more.

2   Notes: Both wild-caught mackerel from the Atlantic and farmed rainbow trout from the U.S. are considered best choices for the environment, according to seafoodwatch.org. For this recipe, you'll need whole mackerel (or rainbow trout) that has been cleaned, butterflied and the heads removed (tails left on). Availability of whole mackerel (or trout) varies, but most fish markets or fish departments at large supermarkets can order and clean the fish for you. Call ahead to make sure you get what you're looking for. Korean chile paste (also called hot pepper paste, gochujang or kochujang) is a fermented spicy condiment made from red chiles, soybeans and salt. Find it in Korean or Asian markets or online from koamart.com. Annie Chun, a widely distributed national

brand of Asian foods, has recently launched their own bottled gochujang sauce that is becoming increasingly available in large supermarkets. It keeps indefinitely in the refrigerator. To make a substitute for Korean chile paste, combine 2 tablespoons white miso, 2 tablespoons Asian-style chile sauce, such as sriracha, and 2 teaspoons molasses. Tip: To oil a grill rack, oil a folded paper towel, hold it with tongs and rub it over the rack. (Do not use cooking spray on a hot grill.)

3   Fish on foil: Fish that flakes easily requires a delicate touch to flip on the grill. If you want to skip turning it over when grilling, measure a piece of foil large enough to hold the fish and coat it with cooking spray. Grill the fish on the foil (without turning) until it flakes easily and reaches an internal temperature of 145°F.

4   People with celiac disease or gluten-sensitivity should use soy sauces that are labeled "gluten-free," as soy sauce may contain wheat or other gluten-containing sweeteners and flavors.

Nutrition Info

221 calories; 7 g fat(1 g sat); 0 g fiber; 4 g carbohydrates; 34 g protein; 12 mcg folate; 87 mg cholesterol; 0 g sugars

DAY 3

BREAKFAST

Golden Milk Chia Seed Pudding

Prep/Cook Time: 6 hrs, Servings:4

Ingredients

- 4 cups full-fat coconut milk
- 3 T honey
- 1 t vanilla extract
- 1 t ground turmeric
- 1/2 t ground cinnamon
- 1/2 t ground ginger
- 1/2 cup chia seeds
- 3/4 cup coconut yogurt, for topping
- 1 cup fresh mixed berries, for garnishing
- 1/4 cup toasted coconut chips, for garnishing

Instructions

1. Combine the coconut milk, honey, vanilla extract, turmeric, cinnamon, and ground ginger together in a large mixing bowl. Mix well to combine, resulting in a vibrant yellow li q uid.
2. Add in the chia seeds, then mix well and set aside for 5 minutes. When ready, stir it around once more.
3. Cover the bowl and let it chill in the refrigerator for at least 6 hours or overnight. This will allow the chia seeds to plump and give the mixture a thick pudding consistency.
4. Divide the chia seed pudding evenly between 4 serving glasses, then top with a dollop of coconut yogurt. Garnish with mixed berries and toasted coconut chips.

Nutrition Info

Calories: 353kcal, Carbohydrates: 10g, Protein: 53g, Fat: 10g,

Saturated Fat: 3g

LUNCH

Sheet Pan Honey Balsamic Salmon with Brussels Sprouts

Prep/Cook Time: 30 mins, Servings: 4

Ingredients

- 4-6oz salmon filets (skin on)
- 16 oz. brussels sprouts, halved
- 1 bunch on asparagus, trimmed and cut in half
- 16 oz. bag of baby potatoes
- 1/2 red onion, cubes
- 1 cup cherry tomatoes
- 2 tablespoons olive oil
- 2 tablespoons honey
- 3 tablespoons balsamic vinegar
- 1 tablespoon dijon mustard
- 1 garlic clove, minced
- 1 teaspoon fresh thyme
- 1/2 teaspoon sea salt

Instructions

1   Preheat oven to 450.
2   In a small bowl, add honey, balsamic vinegar, dijon mustard, garlic, fresh thyme, and salt. Using a whisk, mix together to combine. Set aside.
3   To a large bowl, add brussels sprouts, asparagus, baby potatoes, red onion, cherry tomatoes and olive oil. Add 3 tablespoons of the honey balsamic mixture.
4   Using your hands, toss all of the vegetables to coat them with

the sauce. Spread vegetables out on baking sheet in a single layer.

5   Bake for 10 minutes. Remove from oven.

6   Place salmon filets, skin side down, on top of the vegetables 1? apart. Brush the salmon with the honey balsamic mixture.

7   Place baking sheet back in the oven and bake another 10 minutes.

8   After that switch to broiler HIGH for 3-4 minutes to brown up the top of the salmon. Remove from oven and serve.

Nutrition Info

Calories: 488, Sugar: 15 g, Sodium: 697 mg, Fat: 12 g, Saturated Fat: 2 g, Carbohydrates: 57 g

----

DINNER

Spicy Sweet Potato Black Bean Burgers with avocado-cilantro crema + sprouts

Prep/Cook Time: 1 hour 5 mins, Servings: 6

Ingredients

- 1/2 cup quinoa
- 1 can black beans, rinsed and drained
- 1 large sweet potato
- 1/2 cup diced red onion
- 2 cloves garlic, minced
- 1/2 cup chopped cilantro
- 1/2 jalapeno, seeded and diced
- 1 teaspoon cumin
- 2 teaspoons spicy cajun seasoning
- 1/4 gluten free oat flour (regular oat flour or oat bran will work) salt and pepper, to taste

- olive oil or coconut oil, for cooking
- whole grain hamburger buns (gluten free, if desired) Sprouts
- For Avocado-Cilantro Crema:
- 1/2 large ripe avocado, diced
- 1/4 cup low-fat sour cream or plain greek yogurt
- 2 tablespoons chopped cilantro
- 1 teaspoon lime juice
- dash of hot sauce, if desired salt, to taste

Instructions

1   **To cook quinoa:** Rinse quinoa with cold water in mesh strainer. In a medium saucepan, bring 1 cup of water to a boil. Add in q uinoa and bring mixture to a boil. Cover, reduce heat to low and let simmer for 15 minutes or until q uinoa has absorbed all of the water. Remove from heat and fluff q uinoa with fork; place in large bowl and set aside to cool for about 10 minutes. You should have about 1 1/2 cups of quinoa.

2   Poke sweet potato several times with a fork and place in microwave for about 3-4 minutes or until it is soft and cooked thoroughly. Do not overcook or the sweet potato will harden. Alternatively you can roast the sweet potatoes in the oven at 400 degrees F for 30 minutes or until fork tender. Remove skin when done cooking and cooled.

3   In bowl of food processor, add beans, cooked sweet potato, red onion, cilantro, garlic, cumin, cajun seasoning, and pulse until almost smooth, scraping down the sides of the processor when necessary. Transfer mixture to bowl and combine with cooked q uinoa. Add salt and pepper to taste - and possibly more cajun seasoning if you'd like. Mix in oat bran/oat flour, but only enough so that you are able to shape patties. (You shouldn't need more than 1/3 cup).

4   Divide into 6 patties (about 1/2 cup each) and place on parchment paper on baking sheet; refrigerate for at least 30

minutes to help patties bind together.

5   **To make avocado-cilantro crema:** In bowl of food processor, place sour cream, diced avocado, cilantro, and lime juice. Process until smooth. Add salt to taste. Place in fridge until ready to serve burgers.

6   **To cook burgers:** Heat skillet over medium-high heat. Spray pan with coconut/olive/ canola oil cooking spray. Place in skillet and pan-fry about 3-4 minutes on each side, or until golden brown. Serve with buns, sprouts, crema and desired toppings.

Nutrition Info

Calories: 206, Fat: 6g, Carbohydrates: 33.9g, Sugar: 3.1g, Fiber: 7.2g, Protein: 7.9g

DAY 4

BREAKFAST

Tropical Carrot, Ginger, and Turmeric Smoothie

Prep Time: 5 mins, Servings 2 cups

Ingredients

- 1 blood or navel orange, peel and white pith removed
- 1 large carrot, scrubbed, coarsely chopped
- 1/2 cup frozen mango chunks
- 2/3 cup coconut water
- 1 tablespoon shelled raw hemp seeds
- 3/4 teaspoon finely grated peeled ginger
- 1 1/2 teaspoons finely grated peeled turmeric
- Pinch of cayenne pepper
- Pinch of kosher salt

Instructions

1   Using smoothie or ice crush setting, purée orange, carrot, mango, coconut water, hemp seeds, ginger, turmeric, cayenne, salt, and 1/2 cup ice in a blender until smooth.

Nutrition Info

Calories 234 Calories from Fat 173, Fat 19.18g, Carbohydrates 6.95g, Fiber 3.08g, Protein 7.54g

----

LUNCH

Miso Soup

Prep/Cook Time: 30 mins, Servings 2

Ingredients

For the dashi

- 2 cups water (or substitute 2 cups water, chicken broth, or vegetable broth)
- 1 (2-inch) piece kombu (dried black kelp)
- 1/2 cuploosely packed dried bonito flakes (katsuobushi), optional

For the miso soup:

- 4 ounces silken or firm tofu, drained
- 1 to 2 medium scallions
- 2 tablespoons red or white miso paste

Instructions

2. **Make the dashi:** Combine the water and kombu in a 1-quart saucepan over medium heat. Remove the kombu just as the water starts to come to a boil. Add the bonito flakes, if using, and let the water come to a rapid simmer. Simmer for about 1 minute, then remove the pan from heat and let the bonito steep for an additional 5 minutes. Strain the bonito from the dashi. Add additional water if necessary to make 2 cups. Alternatively, substitute 2 cups water, chicken broth, or vegetable broth.

3. Prepare the tofu and scallions. Cut the tofu into very small cubes, 1/4-inch to 1/2-inch on each side. Slice the scallions very thinly.

4. Bring the broth to a rapid simmer. Pour the dashi or broth back into the saucepan and bring to a rapid simmer over medium-

high heat.

5   Mix the miso with 1/2 cup hot broth. Place the miso in a small ramekin or measuring cup. Scoop out about 1/2 cup of the broth and pour it over the miso. Whisk with a fork or whisk until the miso is entirely dissolved in the water and no lumps remain.

6   Pour the miso into the broth. Pour the dissolved miso into the simmering broth.

7   Add the tofu. Reduce the heat to medium-low and add the tofu to the miso. Simmer just enough to warm the tofu, 1 to 2 minutes. Do not boil the miso once the tofu has been added.

8   Add the scallions. Just before serving, scatter the scallions over the top of the soup. Serve in individual bowls. Pour the miso into individual bowls and serve. Miso is best when served fresh. It will settle a bit as it sits in the broth; whisk briefly with chopsticks or a spoon to mix the soup again.

Nutrition Info

Calories 123, Fat 6 g, Saturated 0.9 g, Carbs 8.5 g, Fiber 2.6 g, Sugars 1.4 g

----

DINNER

One Pan Lemon Herb Salmon and Zucchini

Prep/Cook Time: 35 minutes, 4 servings

Ingredients:

- 4 zucchini, chopped
- 2 tablespoons olive oil
- Kosher salt and freshly ground black pepper, to taste

For the salmon

- tablespoons brown sugar, packed

- 2 tablespoons freshly squeezed lemon juice
- 1 tablespoon Dijon mustard
- 2 cloves garlic, minced
- 1/2 teaspoon dried dill
- 1/2 teaspoon dried oregano
- 1/4 teaspoon dried thyme
- 1/4 teaspoon dried rosemary
- Kosher salt and freshly ground black pepper, to taste
- 4 (5-ounce) salmon fillets
- 2 tablespoons chopped fresh parsley leaves

Instructions:

1. Preheat oven to 400 degrees F. Lightly oil a baking sheet or coat with nonstick spray.
2. In a small bowl, whisk together brown sugar, lemon juice, Dijon, garlic, dill, oregano, thyme and rosemary; season with salt and pepper, to taste. Set aside.
3. Place zucchini in a single layer onto the prepared baking sheet. Drizzle with olive oil and season with salt and pepper, to taste. Add salmon in a single layer and brush each salmon filet with herb mixture.
4. Place into oven and cook until the fish flakes easily with a fork, about 16-18 minutes. Serve immediately, garnished with parsley, if desired.

Nutrition Info

Calories 265, Sugars 9.5g, Protein 18.1g

DAY 5

BREAKFAST

Nutty Choco-Nana Paleo Pancakes

Prep/Cook Time: 20 mins, Servings:10 pancakes

Ingredients

For the Chocolate Sauce:

- 1/4 coconut oil, melted
- 4 T raw cacao powder

For the Pancakes:

- 2 large eggs
- 2 ripe bananas
- 2 T raw cacao powder
- 2 T creamy almond butter
- 1 t pure vanilla extract
- 1/8 t salt
- Coconut oil, for greasing

Instructions

1 **For the Chocolate Sauce:** Melt the coconut oil first and stir in the cacao powder. Mix until fully combined and set aside.

2 For the Pancakes: Preheat a large skillet to medium-low heat and add a tablespoon of coconut oil for greasing.

3 Place all pancake ingredients into a food processor (or blender) and pulse on high until smooth.

4 Using a 1/4 cup measuring cup, scoop out the batter and pour onto the skillet to form one pancake. Cook for five minutes and then carefully flip over to cook for another two minutes. Repeat this process until you have cooked 10 pancakes and the batter is gone. Transfer the pancakes onto a wire baking

rack to cool for five minutes before serving.

5   Keep pancakes in the refrigerator up to five days or in the freezer up to 30 days.

Nutrition Info

Calories 157, Calories from Fat 117, Carbohydrates 10.5g, Fiber 2.6g, Protein 3.9g

----

LUNCH

Shrimp Bok Choy and Turmeric Soup

Prep/Cook Time: 50 mins, Servings: 4

Ingredients

- 1 tablespoon Extra Virgin Olive Oil
- 1 large Onion, chopped
- 6 Garlic Cloves, minced
- 1 1/2 teaspoon Salt, plus additional for serving
- 1 teaspoon Ground Black Pepper, plus additional for serving (optional for AIP)
- 1 teaspoon Turmeric
- 6 cups Chicken Broth
- 2 Carrots, sliced
- 1 pound Shitake Mushrooms, stems removed and sliced into 1/2 inch pieces
- 6 heads Baby Bok Choy, bottoms chopped off
- 1 pound Shrimp

Instructions

1   Heat the oil in a stock pot or dutch oven over medium heat.
2   Add onions and garlic then sauté for 5 minutes or until translucent.

3   Add in salt, pepper, turmeric, chicken broth, carrots and mushrooms then bring to a boil Reduce heat and then let simmer, covered for 20 minutes.

4   Add bok choy and shrimp in the last 5 minutes of cooking. Add salt and pepper to taste then serve.

Nutrition Info

Calories 482, Potassium 386mg, Carbohydrates 3g, Sugar 1g, Protein 16g

----

DINNER

Roasted Cauliflower & Potato Curry Soup

Prep/Cook Time 1 h 30m, 8 servings

Ingredients

- 2 teaspoons ground coriander
- 2 teaspoons ground cumin
- 1 1/2 teaspoons ground cinnamon
- 1 1/2 teaspoons ground turmeric
- 1 1/4 teaspoons salt
- 3/4 teaspoon ground pepper
- 1/8 teaspoon cayenne pepper
- 1 small head cauliflower, cut into small florets (about 6 cups)
- 2 tablespoons extra-virgin olive oil, divided
- 1 large onion, chopped
- 1 cup diced carrot
- 3 large cloves garlic, minced
- 1 1/2 teaspoons grated fresh ginger
- 1 fresh red chile pepper, such as serrano or jalapeño, minced, plus more for garnish
- 1 (14 ounce) can no-salt-added tomato sauce

- 4 cups low-sodium vegetable broth
- 3 cups diced peeled russet potatoes (1/2-inch)
- 3 cups diced peeled sweet potatoes (1/2-inch)
- 2 teaspoons lime zest
- 2 tablespoons lime juice
- 1 (14 ounce) can coconut milk
- Chopped fresh cilantro for garnish

Instructions

1 Preheat oven to 450°F. Combine coriander, cumin, cinnamon, turmeric, salt, pepper and cayenne in a small bowl. Toss cauliflower with 1 tablespoon oil in a large bowl, sprinkle with 1 tablespoon of the spice mixture and toss again. Spread in a single layer on a rimmed baking sheet. Roast the cauliflower until the edges are browned, 15 to 20 minutes.

2 Set aside. Meanwhile, heat the remaining 1 tablespoon oil in a large pot over medium- high heat.

3 Add onion and carrot and cook, stirring often, until starting to brown, 3 to 4 minutes. Reduce heat to medium and continue cooking, stirring often, until the onion is soft, 3 to 4 minutes. Add garlic, ginger, chile and the remaining spice mixture.

4 Cook, stirring, for 1 minute more. Stir in tomato sauce, scraping up any browned bits, and simmer for 1 minute. Add broth, potatoes, sweet potatoes, lime zest and juice.

5 Cover and bring to a boil over high heat. Reduce heat to maintain a gentle simmer and cook, partially covered and stirring occasionally, until the vegetables are tender, 35 to 40 minutes.

6 Stir in coconut milk and the roasted cauliflower. Return to a simmer to heat through. Serve garnished with cilantro and chiles, if desired.

7 To make ahead: Refrigerate for up to 5 days.

Nutrition Info

272 calories; 15 g fat(10 g sat); 7 g fiber; 33 g carbohydrates; 5 g protein; 74 mcg folate; 0 mg cholesterol; 8 g

DAY 6

BREAKFAST

Sweet Potato Cranberry Breakfast Bars

Prep/Cook Time:1 hr 30 mins, Servings:16 bars

Ingredients

- 1 1/2 cups sweet potato purée
- 1/4 cup water
- 2 T coconut oil, melted
- 2 T maple syrup
- 2 eggs
- 1 cup almond meal
- 1/3 cup coconut flour
- 1 1/2 t baking soda
- 1 cup fresh cranberries

Instructions

1   Preheat the oven to 350°F.
2   In a large mixing bowl, combine the sweet potato purée, water, melted coconut oil, maple syrup, and eggs. Stir until combined.
3   In another bowl, sift the almond meal, coconut flour, and baking soda together, and mix well.
4   Add the dry ingredients to the sweet potato mixture and mix well.
5   Grease a 9-inch square baking pan with coconut oil and line the bottom with parchment paper.
6   Transfer the batter to the prepared baking pan and use a wet spatula to smooth out the top and to fill out the corners. Press the cranberries on top.
7   Bake for 30 to 40 minutes or until a toothpick inserted in the

middle comes out clean. Let it cool completely before removing from the pan and slicing into squares.

Nutrition Info

Calories 422, Fat 20g, Protein 17g

LUNCH

Chickpea and Vegetable Coconut Curry

Prep/Cook Time: 30 min, 4 servings

Ingredients

- 1 tablespoon extra-virgin olive oil
- 1 red onion, thinly sliced
- 1 red bell pepper, thinly sliced
- 1 tablespoon fresh ginger, minced
- 3 garlic cloves, minced
- 1 small head cauliflower, cut into bite-size florets
- 2 teaspoons chile powder
- 1 teaspoon ground coriander
- 3 tablespoons red curry paste
- One 14-ounce can coconut milk
- 1 lime, halved
- One 28-ounce can cooked chickpeas
- 1 1/2 cups frozen peas
- Salt and freshly ground black pepper
- Steamed rice, for serving (optional)
- 1/4 cup chopped fresh cilantro
- 4 scallions, thinly sliced

Instructions

1   In a large pot, heat the olive oil over medium heat. Add the

onion and bell pepper, and sauté until nearly tender, 4 to 5 minutes. Add the ginger and garlic, and sauté until fragrant, about 1 minute.

2   Add the cauliflower and toss well to combine. Stir in the chile powder, coriander and red curry paste, and cook until the whole mixture darkens slightly, 1 minute.

3   Stir in the coconut milk and bring the mixture to a simmer over medium-low heat. Cover the pot and continue to simmer until the cauliflower is tender, 8 to 10 minutes.

4   Remove the lid and squeeze lime juice into the curry, stirring well to combine. Add the chickpeas and peas, season with salt and pepper, and bring the mixture back to a simmer.

5   Serve with rice, if desired. Garnish each portion with 1 tablespoon cilantro and 1 tablespoon scallions.

Nutrition Info

665 calories, 31g fat, 80g carbs, 26g protein, 17g sugars

DINNER

Garlic Roasted Salmon & Brussels Sprouts

Prep/Cook Time 45 m, 6 servings

Ingredients

- 14 large cloves garlic, divided
- 1/4 cup extra-virgin olive oil
- 2 tablespoons finely chopped fresh oregano, divided
- 1 teaspoon salt, divided
- 3/4 teaspoon freshly ground pepper, divided
- 6 cups Brussels sprouts, trimmed and sliced
- 3/4 cup white wine, preferably Chardonnay
- 2 pounds wild-caught salmon fillet, skinned, cut into 6 portions
- Lemon wedges

Instructions

1   Preheat oven to 450°F. Mince 2 garlic cloves and combine in a small bowl with oil, 1 tablespoon oregano, 1/2 teaspoon salt and 1/4 teaspoon pepper. Halve the remaining garlic and toss with Brussels sprouts and 3 tablespoons of the seasoned oil in a large roasting pan. Roast, stirring once, for 15 minutes. Add wine to the remaining oil mixture. Remove the pan from oven, stir the vegetables and place salmon on top. Drizzle with the wine mixture. Sprinkle with the remaining 1 tablespoon oregano and 1/2 teaspoon each salt and pepper. Bake until the salmon is just cooked through, 5 to 10 minutes more. Serve with lemon wedges.

Nutrition info:

334 calories; 15 g fat(3 g sat); 3 g fiber; 10 g carbohydrates; 33 g protein

DAY 7

BREAKFAST

Paleo Turmeric Scones

Prep/Cook Time: 35 min, Servings: 6 servings

Ingredients

- 1 1/3 cup almond flour
- 1 cup almonds
- 1/4 cup arrowroot flour
- 1 tbsp coconut flour
- 1 tsp turmeric
- 1/2 tsp black pepper
- Pinch salt
- 1 egg
- 1/4 cup red palm oil
- 3 tbsp maple syrup
- 1 tsp vanilla extract

Instructions

2. Preheat oven to 350°F.
3. Roughly chop almonds in a food processor. Mix chopped almonds with the rest of the dry ingredients, fluff with a fork.
4. Whisk the egg, oil, syrup, and vanilla in a small bowl, add to the dry ingredients. Mix until thoroughly combined, then transfer the dough to a cutting board or countertop covered with plastic wrap. Pat into the round shape approximately an inch thick, then cut into sixths.
5. Bake in the preheated oven for 15-20 minutes or until a tester inserted into the center comes out clean.

Nutrition Info

Calories: 342kcal, Carbohydrates: 8g, Protein: 31g, Fat: 20g,

Saturated Fat: 5g, Cholesterol: 128mg

LUNCH

Kale Pesto Bulgur Salad Recipe

Prep/Cook Time: 30 mins, Servings 4-6

Ingredients

- 1 1/2 cups bulgur
- 1 tsp. kosher salt, divided, plus more to taste
- 1 pint grape tomatoes, halved
- 1/2 pound green beans, trimmed and cut into bite-sized pieces
- 1/4 cup plus 3 Tbsp. sliced almonds, toasted, plus more for garnish
- 1 garlic clove
- 1 cup stemmed and thinly sliced lacinato kale (from about 1/2 bunch)
- 1/2 cup packed basil leaves
- 1/4 packed flat-leaf parsley
- 3 Tbsp. sliced almonds
- 1/4 cup extra-virgin olive oil
- 1/4 cup lemon juice (from about 2 lemons)
- 1/2 tsp. kosher salt
- 1/4 tsp. ground black pepper

Instructions

To make salad:

1   In a large bowl, soak bulgur and 1/2 tsp. salt in 3 cups water overnight. Drain, if needed. (Alternatively, bring 3 cups water to a boil, then pour over bulgur in a heatproof bowl, cover, and let sit 25 minutes. Drain and let cool to room temperature.)

To make pesto:

2   In a food processor fitted with a metal blade, pulse garlic until chopped. Add kale, basil, parsley, and 1/4 cup almonds and pulse again until finely chopped. Add oil, lemon juice, remaining 1/2 tsp. salt, and pepper and puree until smooth.

3   Transfer pesto to bowl with bulgur. Add tomatoes, green beans, and remaining 3 Tbsp. almonds and toss well to combine. Garnish with additional almonds and serve.

Nutrition Info

Calories 444 Calories from Fat 343, Fat 40g, Saturated Fat 18g, Cholesterol 120mg, Sodium 779mg, Protein 17g

----

DINNER

Baked Tilapia Recipe with Pecan Rosemary Topping

Prep/Cook Time 33 mins, Servings 4

Ingredients

- 1/3 cup chopped raw pecans
- 1/3 cup whole wheat panko breadcrumbs
- 2 tsp chopped fresh rosemary
- 1/2 tsp coconut palm sugar or brown sugar
- 1/8 tsp salt
- 1 pinch cayenne pepper
- 1 1/2 tsp olive oil
- 1 egg white
- (4 oz. each) tilapia fillets

Instructions

1   Preheat oven to 350 degrees F.

2   In a small baking dish, stir together pecans, breadcrumbs,

rosemary, coconut palm sugar, salt and cayenne pepper. Add the olive oil and toss to coat the pecan mixture.

3   Bake until the pecan mixture is light golden brown, 7 to 8 minutes.

4   Increase the heat to 400 degrees F. Coat a large glass baking dish with cooking spray.

5   In a shallow dish, whisk the egg white. Working with one tilapia at a time, dip the fish in the egg white and then the pecan mixture, lightly coating each side. Place the fillets in the prepared baking dish.

6   Press the remaining pecan mixture into the top of the tilapia fillets. Bake until the tilapia is just cooked through, about 10 minutes. Serve.

Nutrition Info

Calories 222.4 cal, Calories from fat 90, Total Fat 10.8g, Sodium 153.3mg, Carbohydrate 6.7g, Dietary Fiber 1.6g, Sugars 0.4g, Protein 26.8g

DAY 8

BREAKFAST

Chocolate Avocado Blueberry Muffins

Prep/Cook Time: 28 mins, Servings: 9 muffins

Ingredients

- 2 large eggs, room temperature
- 1 small avocado, ripe
- 1/3 cup coconut sugar
- 1/4 t salt
- 1/4 cup raw cacao powder + 1 T 2 t baking powder
- 2 T coconut flour
- 1 cup almond flour
- 1/2 cup unsweetened almond milk
- 1/4 cup fresh blueberries
- 2 T dark chocolate chips

Instructions

1. Preheat oven to 375°F. Prepare a muffin tin with muffin liners or grease with coconut oil.

2. Place eggs, avocado, sugar and salt in a blender with 1 tablespoon of cacao powder. Blend on high until avocado is fully broken down and the mixture resembles a smooth pudding.

3. In a small bowl, sift together 1/4 cup cocoa powder, baking powder, coconut flour and almond flour.

4. Add the almond milk to the li q uid mixture, then slowly fold in dry ingredients. Mix just until combined - don't overmix!

5. Fold in blueberries and chocolate chips.

6. Transfer batter to prepared muffin tin, dividing the batter evenly among 9 cavities.

7   Bake for 18 minutes or until a toothpick inserted into the center of a muffin comes out clean.

8   Remove the muffins from the tin and transfer to a wire baking rack to cool. Store in the refrigerator for one week or in the freezer for up to one month.

Nutrition Info

Calories 245, Total Fat 23g, Carbohydrates 2g, Protein 4g

LUNCH

Turkey Taco Lunch Bowls

Prep/Cook Time 1 hr 10 mins, Servings: 4

Ingredients

Rice

- 3/4 cup uncooked brown rice
- 1/8 tsp salt
- zest of 1 lime

Turkey

- 3/4 lb lean ground turkey
- 2 tablespoons taco seasoning of choice

Salsa

- 1 pint cherry tomatoes q uartered
- 1 jalapeno minced
- 1/4 cup red onion minced juice from
- 1/2 a lime
- 1/8 tsp salt

Other

- one 12 oz/341 mL can corn kernels drained & rinsed

- 1/4 cup shredded cheese cheddar or mozzarella

Instructions

1 Cook brown rice according to package Instructions, adding the lime zest and salt to the cooking water.
2 Cook turkey over medium heat, tossing in the taco seasoning and breaking it up as you cook. Cook for 10 or so minutes, until cooked through.
3 Combine all salsa ingredients and toss together.

To assemble lunch bowls:

1 -1/4 portion of cooked rice (roughly 1/2 cup)
2 -1/2 cup corn kernels
3 -1/2 cup cooked taco meat
4 -1/4 portion of salsa (just over ½ cup)

Nutrition Info

Calories: 387kcal, Carbohydrates: 42g, Protein: 23g, Fat: 10g, Saturated Fat: 3g

----

DINNER

Crunchy Fresh Broccoli Quinoa Salad

Prep/Cook Time: 25 mins, Servings 2-4

Ingredients

- 1 head broccoli, broken into small florets (about 2 cups)
- 2 cups kale, white parts removed and chopped
- 1/2 small red onion (about 1/2 cup), finely diced
- 1 cucumber, peeled, seeded and diced (about 1 3/4 cups)
- 2 cups seedless red grapes, cut into fourths
- 1/2 cup slivered almonds
- 1 cup cooked quinoa (1/3 cup dry), cooled

- 2 teaspoons apple cider vinegar
- 2 tablespoons vegan mayonnaise
- 1 tablespoon agave nectar
- 1 1/2 tablespoons lemon juice
- 1 teaspoon poppy seeds
- 1/2 teaspoon ground sea salt
- 1/4 teaspoon freshly ground black pepper

Instructions

1. Prepare and chop all ingredients.
2. Add broccoli, kale, red onion, cucumber, grapes, almonds, and q uinoa to a large bowl. In a small bowl, combine apple cider vinegar, mayonnaise, agave, lemon juice, poppy seeds, salt, and pepper. Stir with a spoon or whisk and add the dressing to the vegetable mix. Stir until combined and serve.

Nutrition Info

Calories 142, Fat 12g, Protein 4g, Total Carbs 3g, Fiber 1g

DAY 9

BREAKFAST

Scrambled Eggs With Smoked Salmon Recipe

Prep/Cook Time: 18 Mins., Servings: 2

Ingredients

- 4 eggs;
- 4 slices smoked salmon, chopped
- 2 tbsp. coconut milk
- Fresh chives, finely chopped
- Cooking fat
- Sea salt and freshly ground black pepper;

Instructions

1 In a bowl, whisk the eggs, coconut milk, and fresh chives. Season to taste. Melt some cooking fat in a skillet and add the eggs.
2 Scramble the eggs while cooking.
3 When the eggs start to settle add the smoked salmon and cook for 1 or 2 minutes. Serve with more chives sprinkled on top.

Nutrition Info

Protein: 44g, Carbs: 1g, Fat: 20g / 50%

LUNCH

Lemony Lentil Soup

Prep/Cook Time 1 hour 35 minutes

Ingredients

- 1 tablespoon extra virgin olive oil

- 1 yellow onion, diced
- 1 1/2 cups diced or sliced carrots
- 1 1/2 cups diced celery (1 full head)
- 1 teaspoon salt
- 3 cloves garlic, minced
- 4 teaspoons fresh grated ginger
- 2 1/2 (32 oz.) boxes vegetable broth
- 2 teaspoons dried turmeric
- 2 cups green lentils, rinsed and picked over for stones zest of 1/2 lemon
- juice of 3 small lemons

Instructions

1   Heat oil in a large Dutch oven set over medium heat. Add the onion, carrots, celery, and salt and sauté until softened, about 5 minutes. Add the garlic and ginger and sauté another minute longer. Add the broth, turmeric, and lentils.

2   Reduce heat to low and simmer, partially covered, for 45 minutes. Stir in the lemon zest and juice and simmer another 30 minutes. Add more broth if needed.

Nutrition Info

Calories: 122, Total Fat: 2g, Saturated Fat: 0g

DINNER

Salmon & Fall Vegetables with Bagna Cauda

Prep/Cook Time 40m, 4 servings

Ingredients

- 1 pound fingerling potatoes, halved if large, and/or sweet potato, cut into 1/2-inch-thick wedges

- 1 bunch broccolini, trimmed
- 1 tablespoon extra-virgin olive oil
- 1/2 teaspoon salt, divided
- 1 pound salmon
- 1 small fennel bulb, cut into 1/2-inch-thick wedges, fronds reserved
- 2 medium heads Belgian endive, leaves separated
- 1/2 small head radicchio, cut into 1/2-inch-thick wedges Bagna Cauda
- 1/3 cup extra-virgin olive oil
- 2 cloves garlic, very thinly sliced
- 8 anchovy fillets
- 2 tablespoons sherry vinegar
- 1 tablespoon butter

Instructions

1 Preheat oven to 425°F. Coat a large rimmed baking sheet with cooking spray. Toss potatoes (and/or sweet potato) and broccolini in a large bowl with 1 tablespoon oil and ¼ teaspoon salt. Transfer the potatoes to the prepared baking sheet (leave the broccolini in the bowl). Roast the potatoes, turning once halfway, for 15 minutes. Push the potatoes to the edges of the baking sheet. Place salmon in the middle of the pan and season with the remaining ¼ teaspoon salt. Arrange the broccolini around the salmon. Roast until the vegetables are tender and the salmon is just cooked through, 6 to 10 minutes. Meanwhile, to prepare bagna cauda: Heat oil and garlic in a small saucepan over medium-low heat until the garlic is fragrant, about 2 minutes. Add anchovies and lightly crush until they flake apart. Add vinegar and butter; cook over very low heat, stirring often, for 2 minutes more. Arrange the salmon, potatoes and broccolini with fennel, endive and radicchio on a platter. Garnish with the reserved fennel fronds,

if desired. Serve with the bagna cauda for dipping or drizzling.

Nutrition Info:

537 calories; 30 g fat(6 g sat); 7 g fiber; 35 g carbohydrates; 31 g protein; 82 mcg

DAY 10

BREAKFAST

Smoked Salmon And Spinach Breakfast Recipe

Prep/Cook: 50 min, Servings: 4

Ingredients

- 4 eggs
- 8 oz. smoked salmon, sliced
- 2 russet or sweet potatoes, peeled and diced
- 1/2 onion, sliced
- 1/2 cup mushrooms, sliced
- 2 cups fresh baby spinach
- 1 garlic clove, minced
- 1/2 tsp. onion powder
- 1/2 tsp. garlic powder
- 1/4 tsp. paprika
- 2 tbsp. ghee
- 2 tbsp. olive oil
- Sea salt and freshly ground black pepper

Instructions

2 Preheat oven to 425 F.
3 Dice the potatoes, then drizzle with olive oil, onion powder, garlic powder, paprika, and season to taste.
4 Place the potatoes on a baking dish, and bake in the oven 25 to 30 minutes, turning at the halfway point.
5 Bring a pot of water to a boil over high heat.
6 Add the eggs to the boiling water, turn off the heat and cook 6 to 7 minutes. Drain the water and run cold water over the eggs; peel the eggs and set aside. Melt the ghee over medium-high heat and add the onion and garlic.

7   Cook 1 to 2 minutes, than add the sliced mushrooms.

8   Season everything to taste, and cook until everything is soft, 4 to 5 minutes longer. Add the spinach and cook until wilted, 1 to 2 minutes.

9   Serve the potatoes, topped with the spinach-mushroom mixture, egg, and sliced smoked salmon.

Nutrition Info

Protein: 17g, Carbs: 16g, Fat: 20g

LUNCH

Tuna Salad with Avocado

Prep Time 20 minutes, Servings 6

Ingredients

- 2 cans Genova Seafood Yellowfin Tuna or Albacore Tuna, drained
- 1 cucumber, chopped
- 1/2 red onion, diced
- 1 cup roasted red peppers, chopped
- 1/2 cup pepperocini, diced
- 1/3 cup parsley, finely chopped
- Sundried tomatoes, chopped
- 2 teaspoons capers

Optional:

- 1/4 cup feta cheese
- Optional olives
- 1 14.5 ounce can chickpeas, drained and rinsed
- 1/2 avocado, diced
- Pinch of fine sea salt

- Pinch of black pepper
- Red Wine Vinaigrette
- 2 tablespoons olive oil
- 2 tbsp red wine vinegar
- 1 teaspoon lemon juice
- 1 teaspoon dried parsley
- 1 teaspoon dried oregano
- Pinch fine salt
- Pinch black pepper

Instructions

1   In a large bowl combine all of the salad ingredients. In a small bowl, whisk together dressing ingredients. Pour dressing over ingredients and toss to combine. Taste and adjust spices as desired!

2   Serve over a salad, on a sandwich, with pasta added in, on lettuce wraps, or in 1/2 of an avocado!

Nutrition Info

Calories 244, Fat 20g, Protein 23g, Total Carbs 7g, Fiber 3g Sugar 4g

- - - - - - - - - -

DINNER

Lentil Shrimp Jambalaya

Prep/Cook Time: 45 minutes, Servings: 5

Ingredients

- 1 cup to 1 1/4 cup lentils (uncooked) or 3 cups already cooked
- 3 cups Water or broth to cook lentils if needed
- 170 grams or 1 1/4 cup sliced precooked or uncooked andouille sausage or chicken sausage
- 1 -2 tbsp oil or butter (as needed)

- 2/3 to 1 cup each chopped celery, onion, and bell pepper. Around 2 1/2 c total. The "holy trinity" blend. Feel free to add in extra veggies, like chopped carrots. I did!
- 3 garlic cloves, minced – 1 tsp minced
- 1 jalapeno – sliced (deseed for less spicy)
- 1 cup crushed tomatoes
- 1/2 tsp cajun creole seasoning blend (feel free to add more if you like)
- 2 sprig fresh thyme or 1/2 tsp dried thyme
- pinch of smoked paprika (optional)
- 1 bay leaf
- 14-16 ounces medium shrimp – peeled and deveined
- 1 cup diced okra (fresh or frozen)

FOR THICKER JAMBALAYA MIX IN SLURRY

- 1 tbsp arrowroot starch or cornstarch mixed with equal parts cold water.
- Crushed red pepper flakes to garnish
- Sea salt and freshly-cracked
- black pepper or peppercorns (to taste)

Optional toppings:

- chopped fresh herbs (parsley or cilantro), extra jalapeño, cajun hot sauce

Instructions

1 First, prepare your lentils (if using uncooked). For best results, first rinse lentils thoroughly. If you are using cooked lentils, skip the cooking step below.

2 Lentils: In a large pot, bring 3 cups of li q uid (water or broth) to a boil. Add 1 1/4 cup of rinsed lentils. Cover tightly, reduce heat and simmer for about 15-20 minutes. Drain water from the lentils and set aside in a bowl.

3   In the same pot, add 1 tablespoon oil or butter over medium to medium high heat. NOTE: If you are using uncooked sausage, you may add it here to be browned and then remove. Will need extra oil for sautéeing veggies next. If you are using pre-cooked sausage, then skip the browning and add cooked sliced sausage later with shrimp and lentils.

4   Add your onion, celery, carrots/bell pepper, jalapeño, and garlic. Sauté vegetables on medium to medium-high heat for a few minutes to coat the pan. Or until the onions are slightly browned and fragrant.

5   Next stir in the crushed tomatoes, cooked lentils, cajun spices, smoked paprika, thyme, bay leaf, and stir to combine. Continue cooking until the mixture reaches a simmer. Then reduce heat to medium-low, cover and simmer for about 5 minutes or so. Just to let the flavors release. You will not need to cook long since lentils are already cooked.

6   Lastly, stir in your shrimp and okra. Mix. For thicker jambalaya mix in arrowroot or corn starch slurry. Mix again. Cook on medium, stirring once or twice, for 6-10 minutes or until shrimp or not longer pink. Add your chicken sausage back into the pot and return to low. Remove bay leaf before serving.

7   Serve in bowls and top with red pepper flakes, a dash sea salt and black pepper, and parsley, if desired. I added lots of cajun red hot sauce.

Nutrition Info

Calories 246 Calories from Fat 149, Fat 16.5g, Carbohydrates 1g, Protein 22.5g

DAY 11

BREAKFAST

Savory Indian Pancake

Prep/Cook Time: 20 mins, Servings 4

Ingredients

- oil/fat of choice use enough to shallow fry
- 1/2 cup Almond Flour
- 1/2 cup Tapioca Flour
- 1 cup Coconut Milk canned and full fat
- 1 tsp salt adjust to taste
- 1/2 tsp Kashmiri Chili Powder
- 1/4 tsp Turmeric Powder
- 1/4 tsp freshly ground black pepper
- 1/2 red onion chopped
- 1 handful cilantro leaves chopped
- 1 serrano pepper minced (or adjust to taste)
- 1/2 inch ginger grated

Instructions

Make Batter:

1. Add almond flour, tapioca flour, coconut milk and spices to a bowl - mix together. Then, stir in the onion, cilantro, serrano pepper and ginger.
2. Fry the Pancakes!
3. Heat a saute pan on low-medium heat, add enough oil/fat to coat your pan - then pour ¼ cup of batter onto pan. Spread the mixture out on your pan.
4. Fry this for about 3-4 minutes per side - drizzle a bit more oil on top of the pancake before you flip it. (Stoves vary, so cook until both sides are golden brown).

5. Repeat until batter is done - continue to add oil as needed. Eat with green chutney or paleo ketchup

Nutrition Info

Calories: 441, Fat: 34g, Carbohydrates: 2g, Fiber: 0g, Protein: 32g

----

LUNCH

Glowing Spiced Lentil Soup

Prep/Cook time 35 Minutes, 7 cups (1.65 litres)

Ingredients:

- 1 1/2 tablespoons extra-virgin olive oil
- 2 cups (280 grams) diced onion (1 medium/large)
- 2 large garlic cloves, minced
- 2 teaspoons ground turmeric
- 1 1/2 teaspoons ground cumin
- 1/2 teaspoon cinnamon
- 1/4 teaspoon ground cardamom
- 1 (15-ounce/398 mL) can diced tomatoes, with juices
- 1 (15-ounce/398 mL) can full-fat coconut milk*
- 3/4 cup (140 grams) uncooked red lentils, rinsed and drained
- 3 1/2 cups (875 mL) low-sodium vegetable broth
- 1/2 teaspoon fine sea salt, or to taste Freshly ground black pepper, to taste
- Red pepper flakes or cayenne pepper, to taste (for a kick of heat!)
- 1 (5-ounce/140-gram) package baby spinach
- 2 teaspoons fresh lime juice, or more to taste

Instructions

1 In a large pot, add the oil, onion, and garlic. Add a pinch of

salt, stir, and sauté over medium heat for 4 to 5 minutes until the onion softens.

2   Stir in the turmeric, cumin, cinnamon, and cardamom until combined. Continue cooking for about 1 minute, until fragrant.

3   Add the diced tomatoes (with juices), entire can of coconut milk, red lentils, broth, salt, and plenty of pepper. Add red pepper flakes or cayenne, if desired, to taste. Stir to combine. Increase heat to high and bring to a low boil.

4   Once it boils, reduce the heat to medium-high, and simmer, uncovered, for about 18 to 22 minutes, until the lentils are fluffy and tender.

5   Turn off the heat and stir in the spinach until wilted. Add the lime juice to taste. Taste and add more salt and pepper, if desired. Ladle into bowls and serve with toasted bread and lime wedges.

Nutrition Info

Calories 256, Fat 6g, Protein 1g, Total Carbs 8g, Net Carbs 6g, Fiber 2g, Sugar 4g

----

DINNER

Lentil Shrimp Jambalaya

Prep/Cook Time: 1 hr, Servings 2-4

Ingredients

- 1 tbsp extra-virgin olive oil
- 2 cup grass-fed ground turkey
- 2 cloves garlic — minced
- 1/2 cup onions, diced
- 1 2/3 cup sweet potato, diced

- 1/2 cup homemade tomato sauce Crushed red pepper to taste — optional Salt and pepper
- 2 big bell peppers cut in half
- Feta cheese — don't add cheese if you want to make this recipe paleo-friendly and fresh, chopped parsley.

Instructions

1   Preheat oven to 350F.

2   In a skillet, heat olive oil over medium-high heat.

3   Add ground turkey and garlic. Stir occasionally and cook for about 10 minutes or until the meat is no longer pink. Make sure to break apart the meat with a wood spoon as it cooks.

4   Add onions and cook until onions are golden brown.

5   Add the sweet potato, cover the skillet and cook until they are tender. It takes about 8 minutes.

6   Don't forget to stir occasionally. Add tomato sauce, ground chili pepper, salt, and pepper to taste. If necessary, add more olive oil or a little bit of water to cook the sweet potato.

7   Arrange the peppers in a greased baking dish. The cavity side is facing up. Fill each bell pepper halve with the ground turkey-sweet potato mix.

8   Bake uncovered for about 30 minutes, or until the peppers are cooked and soft. Remove from the oven and garnish with feta and parsley.

Nutrition Info

Calories: 324 Fat: 13.9g Saturated Fat: 4.4g Cholesterol: 88mg, Sodium: 529mg, Carbohydrates: 25.6g, Fiber: 4.4g, Protein: 26.3g

DAY 12

BREAKFAST

Dark Chocolate Orange Chia Pudding

Prep/Cook Time:3 hrs 5 mins, Servings:2

Ingredients

- 1/3 cup chia seeds
- 3 T raw cacao powder
- 1/4 cup orange juice
- 1 T orange zest
- 1 T honey (or maple syrup)
- 1 cup water
- Orange peel, for garnishing (optional)

Instructions

1. In a large bowl, combine the chia seeds, raw cacao powder, orange juice, orange zest, and honey. Mix well.
2. Pour in the water and mix until the cacao powder is fully dissolved.
3. Cover the bowl and let it chill in the refrigerator for at least 3 hours or until the chia seeds have absorbed the li q uid. The chia pudding should be thick.
4. Divide the chia pudding evenly between two glasses, garnish with an orange peel (optional), and serve.

Nutrition Info

Calories: 264, Total Fat: 4g, Saturated Fat: 1g, Sodium: 197mg, Carbohydrates: 6g

----

LUNCH

Winter Fruit Salad with Persimmons, Pears, Grapes, and Pecans

Prep/Cook Time: 25 minutes, Serving: 6 side-dish servings

Ingredients:

- 4 Fuyu persimmons, cut in 1 inch cubes (or enough cut persimmons to make 2 cups)
- 3 Bosch pears, cut in 1 inch cubes (or enough cut pears to make 2 cups)
- 1 cup grapes, cut into halves or fourths if large (I would have used more grapes if I'd had more)
- 3/4 cup pecans, cut into half lengthwise to make slivers Dressing Ingredients:
- 1 T extra virgin olive oil (use a fruity oil for this)
- 1 T peanut oil
- 1 T pomegranate-flavored vinegar (I used pomegranate-flavored red wine vinegar)
- 2 T agave nectar or sweetener of your choice (If you have pomegranate molasses
- I might use white balsamic vinegar and substitute pomegranate molasses for some or all of the agave nectar)
- pinch of salt, to taste

Instructions:

1 Whisk together the dressing ingredients so flavors can blend while you cut the fruit.

2 Cut grapes, persimmons, and pears into same size pieces (about 1 inch size) and place in plastic bowl.

3 Toss fruit with dressing. Just before serving, toss with pecan pieces.

4 Notes:

5   Other fruits such as apples, figs, or pomegranate arils could be used to replace any of these, but you need 5-6 cups of cut fruit.

Nutrition Info

Calories: 270, Total Fat: 18.2g, Carbohydrates: 3g, Fiber: 0.3g, Protein: 22.6g

----

DINNER

Orange-Sesame Salmon with Quinoa & Broccolini

Prep/Cook Time 25 m, 4 servings

Ingredients

- 1 cup quinoa
- 1/2 cup orange juice plus
- 1/3 cup, divided
- 2 scallions, sliced
- 1 bunch broccolini, trimmed
- 1 tablespoon extra-virgin olive oil
- 1/2 teaspoon ground pepper, divided
- 3 teaspoons toasted sesame oil, divided
- 1/4 teaspoon garlic powder
- 4 4-ounce portions wild salmon
- 1 teaspoon black sesame seeds
- 1 tablespoon minced fresh ginger
- 1 tablespoon reduced-sodium tamari
- 1 teaspoon cornstarch

Instructions

1   Prepare q uinoa according to package Instructions, substituting ½ cup orange juice for 1/2 cup water. Remove from heat and stir in scallions. Cover to keep warm. Preheat

oven to 450°F. Line a rimmed baking sheet with foil. Toss broccolini with oil and ¼ teaspoon each salt and pepper in a large bowl. Transfer to the prepared baking sheet. Roast for 8 minutes. Meanwhile, combine 2 teaspoons sesame oil, garlic powder and the remaining 1/4 teaspoon each salt and pepper in a small bowl. Brush the mixture on salmon. Push the broccolini to one side of the pan and place the salmon on the other side. Bake until the salmon is just cooked through, 5 to 8 minutes. Sprinkle the salmon with sesame seeds. Whisk the remaining 1/3 cup orange juice, 1 teaspoon sesame oil, ginger, tamari and cornstarch in a small microwave-safe bowl. Microwave on High for 1 minute. Divide the q uinoa, broccolini and salmon among 4 plates. Drizzle with 2 tablespoons sauce each.

Tips:

Turn leftovers into a salmon & spinach sandwich with wasabi mayo for lunch: Whisk 1 Tbsp. reduced-fat mayonnaise with 1 tsp. wasabi powder. Spread on 1 toasted whole-wheat burger bun. Top with a leftover portion of salmon and ¼ cup baby spinach.

Nutrition info

414 calories; 14 g fat(2 g sat); 4 g fiber; 39 g carbohydrates; 32 g protein; 112 mcg

DAY 13

BREAKFAST

Steel Cut Oats With Kefir And Berries

Cook time: 30 mins, Servings: 4

Ingredients

For the oats:

- 1 cup steel cut oats (look for certified gluten-free if you have a gluten intollerance)
- 3 cups water
- pinch of salt
- For topping (these are all optional, and to-taste):
- fresh or frozen fruit / berries (I used blueberries and raspberries, but any fruit will work)
- a handful of sliced almonds, pepitas, hemp seeds, or other nut/seed (you could even use a little of your favorite granola -- I'm a fan of this Honey & Hazelnut Granola)
- unsweetened kefir, homemade or store-bought
- drizzle of maple syrup, sprinkling of coconut sugar, a few drops of stevia, or any other sweetener you like, to taste

Instructions

1 Add the oats to a small saucepan and place over medium-high heat. Allow to toast, stirring or shaking the pan fre q uently, for 2-3 minutes.

2 Add the water and bring to a boil. Reduce the heat to a simmer, and let cook for about 25 minutes, or until the oats are tender enough for your liking. (The oats will thicken up as they cool -- if you prefer them a bit more porridgy, add a splash more water, or some milk or dairy-free alternative.)

3 Serve with berries, nuts/seeds (or a handful of granola), a

splash of kefir, and any sweetener you like, to taste. Dig in!

Nutrition Info:

Calories: 230, Fat: 30g, Protein: 20g, Net Carbs: 4.75g

LUNCH

Curried Red Lentil and Swiss Chard Soup

Prep/Cook Time: 35 mins, Servings: 6

Ingredients

- 2 tablespoons olive oil
- 1 large onion , thinly sliced
- 5 teaspoons curry powder
- 1/4 teaspoon ground red pepper (cayenne)
- 5 cups vegetable broth
- 1 bunch (1-pound) Swiss chard, tough stalks removed, coarsely chopped
- 2 cups (about 14 ounces) dried red lentils
- 1 can (15-ounce) chickpeas, rinsed and drained
- 1 teaspoon salt
- 6 tablespoons thick Greek yogurt, thinned with
- 2 tablespoons water
- 1 red or green jalapeño chili, stemmed and thinly sliced
- 1 lime, cut into 6 wedges

Instructions

1   Heat oil in large, heavy saucepan over medium heat. Add onion; cook, stirring fre q uently, until lightly golden, about 10 minutes. Stir in curry and red pepper. Add 4 cups broth and chard; increase heat and bring to a boil, stirring until chard is wilted.

2   Stir in lentils and chickpeas. Reduce heat to low, cover, and simmer 16 to 18 minutes, stirring twice, until lentils are tender.

3   Remove from heat. Puree half the soup (about 4 cups) in a blender or food processor; return puree to pot. Stir in remaining 1 cup broth and salt, and warm over low heat 2 minutes.

4   Divide soup among 6 bowls. Drizzle about 1 tablespoon thinned yogurt over each serving. Garnish with a few slices of jalapeño and a lime wedge.

Nutrition Info

Calories: 178, Fat: 12g, Carbohydrates: 6 net grams, Protein: 10g

----

DINNER

Easy Saag Paneer

Prep/Cook Time 25 m, 4 servings

Ingredients

- 8 ounces paneer cheese, cut into 1/2-inch cubes
- 1/4 teaspoon ground turmeric
- 2 tablespoons extra-virgin olive oil, divided
- 1 small onion, finely chopped
- 1 jalapeño pepper, finely chopped (optional)
- 1 clove garlic, minced
- 1 tablespoon minced fresh ginger
- 2 teaspoons garam masala
- 1 teaspoon ground cumin
- 20 ounces frozen spinach, thawed and finely chopped
- 1/4 teaspoon salt
- 2 cups low-fat plain yogurt

Instructions

1   Toss paneer with turmeric in a medium bowl until coated. Heat 1 tablespoon oil in a large nonstick skillet over medium heat. Add the paneer and cook, flipping once, until browned on both sides, about 5 minutes. Transfer to a plate. Add the remaining 1 tablespoon oil to the pan. Add onion and jalapeño (if using) and cook, stirring fre q uently, until golden brown, 7 to 8 minutes. (If the pan seems dry during cooking, add a little water, 2 tablespoons at a time.) Add garlic, ginger, garam masala and cumin. Cook, stirring, until fragrant, about 30 seconds. Add spinach and salt. Cook, stirring, until hot, about 3 minutes. Remove from the heat and stir in yogurt and paneer.

Nutrition Info

382 calories; 24 g fat(12 g sat); 5 g fiber; 19 g carbohydrates; 25 g protein; 223 mcg

DAY 14

BREAKFAST

Red Lentil and Squash Curry Stew

Prep/Cook Time: 22 mins, Servings 4

Ingredients:

- 1 tsp Extra virgin olive oil
- 1 sweet onion, chopped
- 3 garlic cloves, minced
- 1 tbsp good quality curry powder (or more to taste)
- 1 carton broth (4 cups) I used low-sodium
- 1 cup red lentils
- 3 cups cooked butternut squash
- 1 cup greens of choice
- Fresh grated ginger, to taste (optional)
- Kosher salt & black pepper, to taste (I used about 1/2 tsp salt)

Instructions

2 In a large pot, add EVOO and chopped onion and minced garlic. Sautee for about 5 minutes over low-medium heat.

3 Stir in curry powder and cook another couple minutes. Add broth and lentils and bring to a boil. Reduce heat and cook for 10 minutes.

4 Stir in cooked butternut s q uash and greens of choice. Cook over medium heat for about 5-8 minutes. Season with salt, pepper, and add some freshly grated ginger to taste.

Nutrition Info:

Calories: 432, Total Fat 40.4g, Saturated Fat 15.1g, Cholesterol 59mg, Sodium 296.7mg, Protein 30.9g

----

LUNCH

The Ultimate Quinoa-Avocado Bowl

Prep/Cook Time: 45 min, 4 servings

Ingredients

Crispy Kale

- 2 tablespoons extra-virgin olive oil
- 1 bunch lacinato kale, roughly torn
- Salt and freshly ground black pepper

Quinoa

- 2 teaspoons extra-virgin olive oil
- 1 1/4 cups quinoa
- 2 cups chicken broth (or water)
- Salt and freshly ground pepper

Spicy Shrimp & Toppings

- 1 tablespoon extra-virgin olive oil
- 1 pound shrimp, peeled and deveined
- 2 tablespoons hot sauce
- 1 teaspoon ground cumin
- 3/4 teaspoon ground coriander
- Salt and freshly ground black pepper
- 2 California Avocados—peeled, pitted and sliced
- 2 watermelon radishes, thinly sliced

Instructions

1 Make the kale: Preheat the oven to 400°F and line a baking sheet with parchment paper. In a large bowl, toss the olive oil and kale together. Season with salt and pepper.

2 Arrange the kale in an even layer on the baking sheet and roast until very crisp, 15 to 17 minutes.

3   While the kale cooks, make the quinoa: In a medium pot, heat the olive oil over medium heat. Add the q uinoa and toast for about 1 minute, stirring constantly. Add the broth (or water) and bring to a simmer. Simmer until the q uinoa is tender and has absorbed all the liquid. Season with salt and pepper. Set aside.

4   Make the spicy shrimp: In a large skillet, heat the olive oil over medium heat. In a medium bowl, toss the shrimp with the hot sauce, cumin and coriander; season with salt and pepper. Add the shrimp to the skillet and sauté until fully cooked, 4 to 5 minutes.

5   Assemble the bowls: Divide the quinoa among the four bowls and top with a q uarter of the kale and shrimp. Top each bowl with a q uarter of the avocado and watermelon radish slices. Serve immediately.

Nutrition Info

85 calories, 7g fat, 5g carbs, 2g protein, 1g sugars

DINNER

Homemade Green Fried Rice

Prep/Cook Time: 15 mins, Servings 2-4

Ingredients

- 1 tablespoon olive oil
- 1 celery stalk, diced
- 1 small white onion, diced
- 1/2 cup chopped broccoli
- 1 garlic clove, minced
- 2 cups cooked brown rice
- 1/2 cup frozen peas (or fresh if available!)

- 1 tablespoon tamari sauce OR low-sodium soy sauce
- 1 teaspoon honey
- 1/4 teaspoon fresh lemon zest

Instructions

1 Place the olive oil in an oven-safe pan set over medium-high heat. Add the celery, onion, and broccoli to the pan and cook for approximately 2 minutes, just until the onions and celery begin to soften.

2 Add the garlic and rice to the pan, and continue to cook for another 2 minutes.

3 Stir in the frozen peas, tamari and honey. Cook for an additional 3-5 minutes, stirring, until the rice is slightly crisp at the edges.

4 Remove from the heat, and stir in the lemon zest. Serve immediately.

Nutrition Info:

Calories: 234kcal, Carbohydrates: 1g, Protein: 4g, Fat: 4g, Sugar: 1g

DAY 15

BREAKFAST

Roasted cinnamon pear oatmeal

Prep/Cook Time: 1 hr 30 mins, Servings 4

Ingredients

- 3 cups (750g) cooked spaghetti squash
- 4 large (930g) just under ripe red bartlett pears, halved, cored and stalks removed
- 2 tbsp coconut oil, softened but not melted (I use this one)
- 1 tsp powdered cinnamon (I use this one)
- 1+1/4 cups (110g) shredded coconut (I use this one)
- 2+1/2 cups (625ml) coconut milk (I use this one)
- 1 tsp salt (I use this one)

Instructions

The night before:

1. Preheat the oven to 350°F/180°C.
2. Prepare a large s q uash by cutting it in half across the width, scooping out the seeds and putting it cut side down in a roasting pan large enough to hold both halves. Pour a half inch worth of water into the pan and bake for about 45 minutes to an hour. You want the flesh to be nice and soft, beyond that spaghetti stage so if you go over the 45 minute mark, like I often do when I get distracted and end up leaving it for nearly an hour and a half, I wouldn't worry! Carefully remove the piping hot s q uash halves and put them onto plates to cool before popping into the fridge overnight.
3. In a small bowl, mix the coconut oil and cinnamon powder together, ignoring the fact it looks remarkably like

forbidden chocolate sauce, and divide between the pear halves, spooning into and along the wells. Place into a large roasting tin and bake alongside the s q uash for 30 minutes. Baste the pears all over with the juices that have run into the pan, turn them so they are cut side down and continue roasting an extra 15 minutes or until nicely browned, slightly caramelised, smelling fantastic and you can put a knife through them easily. You don't want the pears so soft to the point of falling apart. Set aside to cool before putting into a covered container (along with the juices) and leaving in the fridge overnight.

On 'oatmeal day':

1   Roughly chop three of the pears (six halves) and put them into a large pan along with the squash, shredded coconut, coconut milk and salt. Make sure to add in the coconut/cinnamon that has now set on the bottom of the dish. Mix well and bring to the boil. Immediately turn down to a simmer and cook, stirring fre q uently until piping hot throughout, approx 8-10 minutes. Use an immersion blender to break down the fibres of the s q uash, but leaving it fairly chunky.

2   Serve the oatmeal with reserved pear halves sliced artistically over the top.

Nutrition Info:

Calories: 434, Fat: 28g, Carbohydrates: 4g, Fiber: 1g, Protein: 35g

----

LUNCH

One-Sheet Roasted Garlic Salmon & Broccoli

Prep/Cook Time: 20 mins, Servings 2-4

Ingredients:

- 1 1/2 pounds salmon fillets, skinned and cut into 4 portions
- 2 heads of broccoli, washed and cut into florets (about 4 cups)
- 3 tablespoons avocado oil or melted coconut oil
- 1-2 cloves of garlic, minced and divided
- 1 1/4 teaspoon of sea salt, divided
- 1/2 teaspoon ground black pepper, divided sliced lemon (optional)

Instructions

1 Preheat oven to 450F and line a large baking sheet with parchment paper or a silicon baking mat.

2 Arrange the salmon pieces on the lined baking sheet, leaving a few inches between the portions. Drizzle 1 tablespoon of oil over the fish. Spread the minced garlic cloves evenly over the salmon next. Next, sprinkle the fish with 1/2 teaspoon salt and 1/4 teaspoon ground black pepper. Finally, arrange the sliced lemon (if using) on top of the salmon pieces.

3 Next, combine the clean broccoli florets 2 tablespoons of oil, 3/4 teaspoon sea salt and 1/4 teaspoon ground black pepper in a medium bowl. Toss to evenly coat the florets. Arrange the broccoli on the baking sheet around the salmon pieces.

4 Bake in the oven for 13-15 minutes or until fish is done and the broccoli florets are slightly golden on the ends.

5 Enjoy warm.

Nutrition Info

Calories 354 Calories from Fat 216, Fat 24g, Carbohydrates 2g, Sugar 1g, Protein 42g

----

DINNER

Curried Potatoes with Poached Eggs

Prep/Cook Time: 40 mins, Servings: 4

Ingredients

- 2 russet potatoes (about 2 lbs.)
- 1inch fresh ginger
- 2 cloves garlic
- 1 Tbsp olive oil
- 2 Tbsp curry powder (hot or mild)
- 15 oz can tomato sauce
- 4 large eggs
- 1/2 bunch fresh cilantro (optional)

Instructions

2 Wash the potatoes well, then cut into 3/4-inch cubes. Place the cubed potatoes in a large pot and cover with water. Cover the pot with a lid and bring it up to a boil over high heat. Boil the potatoes for 5-6 minutes, or until they're tender when pierced with a fork. Drain the cooked potatoes in a colander.

3 While the potatoes are boiling, begin the sauce. Peel the ginger with a vegetable peeler or scrape the skin off with the side of a spoon. Use a small holed cheese grater to grate about one inch of ginger (less if you prefer a more subtle ginger flavor). Mince the garlic.

4 Add the ginger, garlic, and olive oil to a large, deep skillet (or a wide based pot). Sauté the ginger and garlic over medium low heat for 1-2 minutes, or just until soft and fragrant. Add the curry powder to the skillet and sauté for

about a minute more to toast the spices.

5   Add the tomato sauce to the skillet and stir to combine. Turn the heat up to medium and heat the sauce through. Taste the sauce and add salt, if needed. Add the cooked and drained potatoes to the skillet and stir to coat in the sauce. Add a couple tablespoons of water if the mixture seems dry or pasty.

6   Create four small wells or dips in the potato mixture and crack an egg into each. Place a lid on the skillet and let it come up to a simmer. Simmer the eggs in the sauce for 6-10 minutes, or until cooked through (less time if runny yolks are desired). Top with chopped fresh cilantro.

Notes

If you don't have a large deep skillet like mine, a wide pot will do the trick. Make sure your skillet or pot has a lid and is big enough to hold the potatoes.

DAY 16

BREAKFAST

Banana Chia Pudding

Prep/Cook Time: 4 hours 5 minutes, 3 servings

Ingredients

- 1 large banana, very ripe
- 1/2 cup chia seeds
- 2 cups any milk (I used unsweetened almond milk)
- 1/2 tsp pure vanilla extract
- 2 tbsp raw honey or maple syrup
- 1 tbsp cacao powder

Mix-ins:

- 1 large banana, sliced
- 2 tbsp chocolate chips
- 2 tbsp cacao nibs

Instructions

1   In a medium bowl, add banana and chia seeds. Mash with a fork until well combined. Add milk and vanilla extract; whisk until well mixed and no lumps appear.
2   Pour half into a glass container and cover. Add maple syrup and cacao powder to remaining half and whisk well. Pour into another container with a lid. Refrigerate both for at least 4 hours or overnight.
3   To serve: in 3 bowls or glasses layer e q ually both chia puddings with mix-ins.

Nutrition Info:

Calories 293, Total Fat 13.7g, Sodium 90.8mg, Total Carbohydrate 39.6g

----

LUNCH

Lentil, Beetroot and Hazelnut Salad
With a Ginger Dressing

Active Time 10 minutes

Prep/Cook Time 10 minutes, Servings 2–3

Ingredients

For the salad:

- 1 cup Puy lentils, rinsed
- 2 3/4 cup filtered water
- Sea salt
- 3 cooked beetroot, cut into small cubes
- 2 spring onions, finely sliced
- 2 tablepoons hazelnuts, roughly chopped
- A handful of fresh mint, roughly chopped
- A handful of fresh parsley, roughly chopped

For the ginger dressing:

- 3/4-inch cube of fresh ginger, peeled and roughly chopped
- 6 tablepoons olive oil
- 1 teaspoon Dijon mustard
- 1 tablespoon apple cider vinegar
- Pinch of sea salt and freshly ground black pepper

Instructions

1 For the lentils, put them in a saucepan, cover with water, bring to a boil the reduce the heat and simmer for about 15–20 minutes, or until all the li q uid has evaporated and the lentils are not mushy and still with a bite.

2 As soon as the lentils are cooked transfer them to a large bowl

and leave to cool.

3   Once the lentils are cool, add the beetroot, spring onions, hazelnuts and herbs and stir until everything is combined.

4   For the dressing, put the ginger, mustard, oil and vinegar in a bowl and, using a hand- held blender, blend until combined.

5   Drizzle the dressing over the salad and serve.

Nutrition Info

Calories 815, Carbohydrates 78g, Fat 46g, Protein 28g, Saturated Fat 6g, Sodium 1486 mg

----

DINNER

Romaine Wedges with Sardines & Caramelized Onions

Prep/Cook Time: 30 m, 4 servings

Ingredients

- 1 tablespoon canola oil
- 1 large sweet onion, sliced
- 1/8 teaspoon salt plus 1/2 teaspoon, divided
- 2 tablespoons balsamic vinegar
- 1/2 cup reduced-fat plain Greek yogurt
- 2 tablespoons low-fat mayonnaise
- 2 tablespoons white-wine vinegar
- 4 teaspoons minced shallot
- 1/4 teaspoon freshly ground pepper
- 2 hearts of romaine, halved lengthwise and cored
- 2 4-ounce cans sardines with bones, packed in olive oil, drained
- 1 cup halved grape or cherry tomatoes

Instructions

1 Place oil, onion and 1/8 teaspoon salt in a small saucepan over medium heat. Cover and cook, stirring occasionally, until the onions are very soft and starting to brown, 12 to 15 minutes. Reduce heat to medium-low if they are browning too much. Stir in balsamic vinegar and simmer, uncovered, until it is reduced to a glaze, 1 to 3 minutes. Whisk yogurt, mayonnaise, white-wine vinegar, shallot, pepper and the remaining ½ teaspoon salt in a small bowl. Divide romaine halves among 4 dinner plates or place on a large platter. Spoon the dressing over the salads. Break sardines into two or three pieces each and divide among the romaine halves. Top with the caramelized onions and tomatoes.

2 Make Ahead Tip: To make ahead: Cover and refrigerate the dressing (Step 2) for up to 2 days.

Nutrition info

202 calories; 10 g fat(2 g sat); 3 g fiber; 13 g carbohydrates; 14 g protein; 169 mcg

DAY 17

BREAKFAST

Anti-Inflammatory Blueberry Smoothie

Prep Time: 5 mins, Servings: 1

Ingredients

- 2 handfuls spinach or leafy greens
- 1 frozen banana
- 2/3 - 1 cup frozen blueberries
- 1 T almond butter
- 1/4 tsp cinnamon
- 1/8 - 1/4 tsp cayenne start light and add as desired
- 1 tsp maca powder optional
- 1/2 cup water
- 1/2 cup unsweetened almond milk

Instructions

1 Combine all ingredients in a high powered blender and blend until smooth. Serve immediately.

Nutrition Info

Calories: 329, Fat: 31g, Carbohydrates: 10g net, Protein: 16g

----

LUNCH

Roasted Red Pepper and Sweet Potato Soup

Prep/Cook Time: 55 minutes, 6 servings

Ingredients

- 2 tablespoons olive oil

- 2 medium onions, chopped
- 1 jar (12 oz) roasted red peppers, chopped, liquid reserved
- 1 can (4 oz) diced green chiles
- 2 teaspoons ground cumin
- 1 teaspoon salt
- 1 teaspoon ground coriander
- 3 – 4 cups peeled, cubed sweet potatoes
- 4 cups vegetable broth
- 2 tablespoons minced fresh cilantro
- 1 tablespoon lemon juice
- 4 oz cream cheese, cubed

Instructions

2   In a large soup pot or Dutch oven, heat the olive oil over medium-high heat. Add the onion and cook until soft. Add in the red peppers, green chiles, cumin, salt and coriander. Cook for 1-2 minutes.

3   Stir in the reserved juice from the roasted red peppers, sweet potatoes and vegetable broth. Bring to a boil, then reduce heat and cover. Cook until the potatoes are tender, 10-15 minutes. Stir in the cilantro and lemon juice. Let the soup cool slightly.

4   Place half of the soup into a blender along with the cream cheese. Process until smooth, then add back into the soup pot and heat through. Season with additional salt, if needed.

Nutrition Info

Calories: 334, Fat: 18g, Carbohydrates: 6g, Protein: 24g

DINNER

Spaghetti Squash Alfredo

Prep/Cook Time: 1 hr 50 mins, Servings 2-4

Ingredients

- 2-3 pound spaghetti squash
- 1 tablespoon olive oil
- 2 garlic cloves, finely minced
- 2 tablespoons brown rice flour OR whole wheat flour OR white flour
- 1 cup low-fat milk
- 1 tablespoon Greek yogurt
- 1/2 cup grated Parmesan cheese
- 1 teaspoon dried thyme
- Salt & pepper to taste

Instructions

1　Preheat your oven to 350 degrees.
2　Using a knife, poke several small holes in the exterior of the s q uash. This will allow some steam to escape the squash while roasting it in the oven—and prevent it from exploding!
3　Place the whole squash on a baking sheet. Bake for approximately 45 minutes to an hour, until the squash is soft to the touch, and water is starting to seep out.
4　Remove from the oven, and allow the squash to come to room temperature before slicing it in half lengthwise. Remove all of the seeds, and any fibrous portions from the center.
5　Meanwhile, make the Alfredo sauce. Place the oil in a saucepan set over medium heat. Add the garlic to the pan, and cook for approximately 2-3 minutes, just until fragrant. Add the flour to the pan, and stir, allowing it to "toast" for a minute or so.

6   Whisk the milk into the pan, incorporating the flour, stirring out any lumps as you go. Bring the milk to a gentle boil. The sauce will thicken as it warms.

7   Once boiling, remove the sauce from the stovetop, stir in the yogurt, Parmesan cheese, and dried thyme. Add salt and pepper to taste.

8   With a fork, gently "shred" the interior of the spaghetti squash halves. It will resemble pasta!. Pour the sauce over each half.

9   Broil the halves, just until bubbling, and the sauce is lightly browned. Serve out of the oven.

Nutrition Info

Calories: 222kcal, Carbohydrates: 2g, Protein: 4g, Fat: 8g, Sodium: 145mg

DAY 18

BREAKFAST

Pineapple Smoothie

Prep/Cook Time: 5 mins, Servings 2-4

Ingredients:

- 1 ½ cups frozen pineapple chunks
- 1 orange, peeled
- 1 cup coconut water
- 1 tablespoon finely-chopped fresh ginger (or 1/4 teaspoon ground ginger)
- 1 teaspoon chia seeds, plus extra for garnishing
- 1 teaspoon McCormick Ground Turmeric
- 1/4 teaspoon ground black pepper

Instructions:

1 Add all ingredients to a blender. Pulse until smooth.
2 Serve immediately, garnished with extra chia seeds if desired.

Nutrition Info

Calories: 120, Fat: 19g, Carbohydrates: 9g, Fiber: 2g, Protein: 13g

----

LUNCH

Turkish Scrambled Eggs

Prep/Cook Time: 35 minutes, Servings 4

Ingredients

- 2 Tbsp. canola or olive oil
- 3 scallions, finely chopped
- 2 large red bell peppers, seeded and finely chopped

- 2 to 4 ripe tomatoes, diced (about 1 pound)
- 1 tsp. crushed red pepper flakes
- 6 eggs, beaten
- 4 ounces crumbled Feta cheese (optional)
- 1/2 tsp. kosher salt
- 1/4 tsp. ground black pepper
- 2 Tbsp. chopped fresh parsley
- Green olives, for garnish (optional)
- 4 whole grain pitas, for serving

Instructions

1   In a medium skillet, heat oil over medium-high heat. Add scallions and cook until soft, about 2 minutes. Add peppers; continue cooking 5 minutes. Add tomatoes and red pepper flakes and sauté until some of the liquid from the tomato starts to evaporate.

2   Add the eggs and Feta (if using), and scramble, stirring constantly, until eggs are fully cooked and coat the vegetables. Season with salt and pepper, adding more to taste. Remove from heat and stir in parsley. Serve with green olives (if using) and whole grain pitas on the side.

Nutrition Info:

346 calories, 21 grams fat, 18 grams protein, 23 grams carbohydrates.

DINNER

Turkey & Quinoa Stuffed Peppers

Prep/Cook Time: 40 mins, Servings 2-4

Ingredients:

- 3 large yellow peppers

- 1.25 lb extra lean ground turkey
- 1 C diced mushrooms
- 1/4 C diced sweet onion
- 1 C chopped fresh spinach
- 2 teaspoons minced garlic
- 1 C (1 8oz can) tomato sauce
- 1 C chicken broth
- 1 C dry quinoa

Instructions:

1   In a small saucepan, start the q uinoa and cook according to package Instructions (usually about 15 minutes).

2   While the quinoa cooks, saute the vegetables in a pan with a little butter or olive oil. Then after about 5 minutes or so, add the ground turkey and garlic to the vegetables. Cook over medium heat. Once the turkey is mostly cooked though, add in the tomato sauce and about half of the chicken broth. Let simmer until the turkey is fully cooked and some of the excess liquid has cooked off.

3   Preheat the oven to 400.

4   While the turkey mixture simmers, prep your bell peppers. Wash the peppers, cut them in half, and remove the stem & seeds. Spray a 9×13 baking pan with cooking spray and place the cut bell peppers in the pan (open side up).

5   Once the q uinoa is done cooking, dump it into the pan with the turkey & vegetables. Stir together. Then, stuff each bell pepper with the mixture. Make sure they are nice & full! If you're opting for cheese, then top with just enough cheese to barely cover the mixture (if you put too much on, it will get super messy in the oven!). Pour the rest of the chicken broth into the base of the pan (so around the peppers, not over them). Turkey & quinoa stuffed yellow peppers

6   Cover with foil and bake at 400 for about 30-35 minutes.

Serve warm & eat up! They are sooooo good!

Nutrition Info

Calories: 346, Total Carbs: 14.41g, Fiber: 6.27g

☆☆☆☆☆

DAY 19

BREAKFAST

Sweet Plantain Waffles

Prep/Cook Time: 30 mins, Servings 2-4

Ingredients

- 2 Cups (2-3 large) pureed medium ripe-ripe plantains
- 2 1/2 Tablespoons coconut oil, melted + more for oiling the waffle maker
- 1 Teaspoon cinnamon
- 1 Teaspoon pure vanilla extract
- 1 Teaspoon apple cider vinegar
- 1/2 Teaspoon sea salt
- 1/2 Teaspoon baking soda

Instructions

1 Heat your waffle iron. (I set the heat to 5 out of a possible 6) Peel the plantains and chop them each into 4 pieces.

2 Place the plantain pieces in a high speed blender and blend until smooth (or as smooth as possible until it becomes too difficult to blend more).

3 Add the oil to the plantains and blend again, now until completely pureed.

4 Add the cinnamon, vanilla and apple cider vinegar to the blender. Blend again on high for a few seconds to mix well.

5 Add the salt and baking soda to the blender. You can blend again to mix or use a spatula to stir the ingredients into the batter by hand.

6 Oil your waffle iron and place? cup of batter into the center of your waffle iron. The amount of batter you use may vary depending on your waffle maker and it's instructions. I have

used a Belgian and classic waffle maker. Both work, but I prefer the classic.

7   Cook until the waffle is browned to your liking, and repeat until the batter is gone. Be sure to keep the waffle maker oiled before each waffle.

8   Transfer the cooked waffles to a wire cooling rack rather than stacking them on a plate as you cook.

9   Serve with maple syrup, fresh fruit and whipped coconut cream!

Nutrition Info

Calories: 348 Calories, Total Carbs: 10.41g, Fiber: 4g, Net Carbs: 6.14g, Protein: 38.38g, Fat: 40.21g

----

LUNCH

Smoked salmon salad with green goddess dressing

Prep/Cook Time: 35 minutes, Servings: 4

Ingredients

- 105g (1/2 cup) French green lentils, rinsed
- 2 baby fennel bulbs, thinly sliced, some fronds reserved
- 130g (1/2 cup) natural yoghurt
- 2 tablespoons chopped fresh continental parsley, plus extra parsley leaves, to serve
- 2 tablespoons chopped fresh chives
- 1 tablespoon chopped fresh tarragon
- 1 tablespoon salted baby capers, rinsed, drained
- 1 teaspoon finely grated lemon rind
- 1/2 red onion, thinly sliced
- 1 tablespoon fresh lemon juice
- Pinch of caster sugar

- 60g baby spinach
- 1/2 avocado, sliced
- 180g sliced salt-reduced smoked salmon

Instructions

1   Cook lentils in a large saucepan of boiling water for 20 minutes or until tender. Drain. Meanwhile, heat a chargrill pan over high heat. Spray fennel slices with oil. Cook for 2 minutes each side or until tender.

2   Process the yoghurt, parsley, chives, tarragon, capers and lemon rind in a food processor until smooth. Season with pepper.

3   Place onion, juice, sugar and a pinch of salt in a bowl. Set aside for 5 minutes. Drain. Combine the lentils, fennel, onion, spinach and avocado in a large bowl. Divide among plates. Top with salmon. Sprinkle with the reserved fennel fronds and extra parsley. Drizzle with the green goddess dressing.

Nutrition Info

Calories: 520kcal, Carbohydrates: 2g, Protein: 45g, Fat: 62g, Saturated Fat: 25g

----

DINNER

Red Cabbage Salad with Blue Cheese & Maple-Glazed Walnuts

Prep/Cook Time: 20 mins, Servings 8

Ingredients

- 1 tablespoon crumbled blue cheese
- 1/4 cup extra-virgin olive oil
- 3 tablespoons red-wine vinegar

- 1 tablespoon Dijon mustard
- 1/4 teaspoon salt
- 1/4 teaspoon freshly ground pepper
- 1 tablespoon extra-virgin olive oil
- 1 teaspoon butter
- 1 cup walnuts
- 1/4 teaspoon salt
- 1/4 teaspoon freshly ground pepper
- 3 tablespoons pure maple syrup
- 8 cups very thinly sliced red cabbage
- 2 scallions, thinly sliced
- 1/3 cup crumbled blue cheese

Instructions

1   To prepare vinaigrette: Combine 1 tablespoon blue cheese, ¼ cup oil, vinegar, mustard, salt and pepper in a mini food processor or blender; process until creamy. To prepare salad: Place a piece of parchment or wax paper near your stove. Heat 1 tablespoon oil and butter in a medium skillet over medium heat. Add walnuts and cook, stirring, for 2 minutes. Add salt and pepper and drizzle in maple syrup. Cook, stirring, until the nuts are well coated and have begun to caramelize, 3 to 5 minutes. Transfer to the paper, spooning any remaining syrup over them. Separate the nuts while they're still warm. Let stand until cool, about 5 minutes. Place cabbage and scallions in a large bowl. Toss with the vinaigrette. Serve topped with blue cheese and the walnuts. Make Ahead Tip: Store glazed walnuts (Step 2) airtight for up to 1 day.

Nutrition info

232 calories; 19 g fat(4 g sat); 2 g fiber; 12 g carbohydrates; 4 g protein

DAY 20

BREAKFAST

Whole30 Sweet Potato Protein Breakfast Bowl

Prep/Cook Time: 5 mins, Servings: 1

Ingredients

- 1 small sweet potato, pre-baked
- 1 serving protein powder*
- 1 small banana, sliced
- 1/4 cup raspberries
- 1/4 cup blueberries

optional toppings

- cacao nibs chia seeds hemp hearts
- favorite nut/seed butter

Instructions

2 Flesh out sweet potato if not done already. In a small bowl, mash sweet potato with fork. Stir in protein powder until combined.

3 Layer in banana slices, raspberries, and blueberries. Top with additional desired toppings and dig in! You can enjoy this bowl warm or cold, your choice!

Nutrition Info:

Calories: 302, Sugar: 24, Fat: 1, Carbohydrates: 54, Fiber: 9, Protein: 23

LUNCH

Life-Changing Loaf of Bread

Prep time: 48 hrs & Cook time: 1 hrs, Servings 4

Ingredients

- 1 cup (135 grams) sunflower seed kernels (not in the shell)
- 1/2 cup (90 grams) flax seeds
- 1/2 cup (65 grams) hazelnuts or almonds
- 1 1/2 cups (145 grams) rolled oats (if making gluten-free, make sure to get certified gluten-free oats)
- 2 tablespoons chia seeds
- 4 tablespoons psyllium seed husks (3 tablespoons if using psyllium husk powder)
- 1 teaspoon fine grain sea salt (add 1/2 teaspoon if using coarse salt)
- 1 tablespoon maple syrup (for sugar-free diets, use a pinch of stevia)
- 3 tablespoons melted coconut oil or ghee
- 1 1/2 cups (350 milliliters) water

Instructions

1 In a flexible, silicon loaf pan or a standard loaf pan lined with parchment, combine all dry ingredients, stirring well. Whisk maple syrup, oil, and water together in a measuring cup. Add this to the dry ingredients and mix very well until everything is completely soaked and dough becomes very thick (if the dough is too thick to stir, add one or two teaspoons of water until the dough is manageable). Smooth out the top with the back of a spoon. Let sit out on the counter for at least 2 hours, or all day or overnight. To ensure the dough is ready, it should retain its shape even when you pull the sides of the loaf pan away from it or lift the parchment.

2   Preheat oven to 350° F / 175° C.

3   Place loaf pan in the oven on the middle rack, and bake for 20 minutes. Remove bread from loaf pan, place it upside down directly on the rack and bake for another 30 to 40 minutes. Bread is done when it sounds hollow when tapped. Let cool completely before slicing.

4   Store bread in a tightly sealed container for up to five days. Freezes well too – slice before freezing for quick and easy toast!

Nutrition Info

Calories: 423kcal, Carbohydrates: 17g, Protein: 42g

DINNER

Deep Dish Falafel Pizza

Prep/Cook Time: 60 mins, Servings 2-4

Ingredients

For the Falafel Crust:
- 3/4 cup cooked chickpeas
- 1/3 cup millet, oats, or flour
- 1 small red onion
- 1 cup fresh mint
- 1 cup fresh coriander
- 2 cloves garlic
- 3 tablespoons tahini
- 3 tablespoons ground chia or flax
- 2 tablespoons cumin
- 2 tablespoons coriander powder

For the Beet Hummus:
- 1/2 cup cooked chickpeas

- 1 small beet, boiled
- 2 tablespoons tahini
- 1 cloves garlic
- Oregano, basil, and other herbs, as desired
- Sliced vegetables, as desired

For the Tahini Cheese Sauce:

- 2 tablespoons tahini
- Nutritional yeast, to taste

Instructions

1 Preheat oven to 390°F. Line a cake pan or deep pie dish with baking paper.

To Make the Base:

1 In a food processor, pulse all crust ingredients, until all ingredients are very combined and have become little pieces.

2 Spread on the bottom and lower sides of cake pan/pie dish. Bake in oven for 20 minutes

To Make the Beet Hummus:

1 In a food processor, pulse all ingredients, until smooth.

2 Remove the beet hummus, add the sliced vegetables to the hummus, and mix When the falafel crust is dry to the touch, remove from oven.

3 Pour the beet hummus on top of the crust and return to the oven for around 40 minutes.

To Make the Cheese Sauce:

1 Mix all ingredients together and drizzle on top of pizza when it has finished baking. Slice and serve.

Nutrition Info

Calories: 350kcal, Carbohydrates: 4g, Protein: 38g, Fat: 46g, Saturated Fat: 11g

☆☆☆☆☆

DAY 21

BREAKFAST

Turmeric Hot Chocolate

Prep/Cook Time: 5 mins, Servings 4

Ingredients

- 1 cup Milk (250ml)
- 1 1/2 tbsp Unsweetened Cocoa Powder
- 1 tsp Ground Turmeric
- 2 tsp Coconut Oil, to help absorb the turmeric
- A Pinch of Black Pepper, to help absorb the turmeric
- A Pinch of Cayenne Pepper
- 2 tsp Honey

Instructions

1 Pour milk in a sauce pan. Add cocoa powder, turmeric and coconut oil. Mix everything with a whisk until combined and bring to a boil.
2 Turn off the heat, add a pinch of black peper and cayenne pepper and give it a stir. Pour in a mug. Let it cool down a bit before adding honey.
3 Serve warm.
4 Recipe Notes
5 Honey can be substituted with sugar, agave syrup or maple syrup.
6 Coconut oil and black pepper are important here as they help your body absorb turmeric.
7 Cayenne pepper can be omitted.

Nutrition Info

Calories 295, Calories from Fat 162, Total Fat 18g, Saturated Fat 13g, Cholesterol 24mg, Total Carbohydrates 29g

----

LUNCH

Smoked Salmon Potato Tartine

Prep/Cook Time: 45 minutes, 2 Servings

Ingredients

Potato Tartine:

- 1 large russet potato, peeled and grated lengthwise
- 2 tablespoons clarified butter (or other neutral flavored oil) salt

Pepper Toppings:

- 4 ounces soft goat cheese, at room temperature
- 1 1/2 tablespoons finely minced chives
- 1/2 garlic clove, finely minced
- zest of half a lemon
- thinly sliced smoked salmon
- 2 tablespoons drained capers
- 2 tablespoons finely chopped red onion
- 1/2 hard boiled egg, finely chopped
- finely minced chives (for garnish)

Instructions:

Assemble Toppings:

1 Combine goat cheese, lemon zest, and garlic in small bowl. Season with salt and pepper to taste. Gently stir in fresh chives. Set aside.

2 Season the chopped red onion and hard-boiled egg with salt.

Prepare Potato Tartine:

1 Working q uickly (as the potato will quickly begin to oxidize),

grate the potato (lengthwise) into a large using the large holes of a grater. Squeeze the potatoes over the sink to remove any excess li q uid. Season generously with salt and pepper and toss.

2   Heat clarified butter in a 8-10 inch non-stick skillet over medium-high heat. Once hot, add the grated potato and shape roughly, using a spatula, into a large circle.

3   Press on the mixture with the back of a spoon to compact it, cover and cook gently for 8-10 minutes or until the bottom is golden brown.

4   Flip carefully to other side and cook for another 8-10 minutes or until golden brown and crispy.

5   Remove to cooling rack and allow to cool until barely lukewarm or room temperature.

Assemble Tartine:

1   Once potato cake has cooled, spread the goat cheese mixture on the top. Layer the smoked salmon directly over this and sprinkle with the red onion, hard-boiled egg, and capers. Garnish with freshly chopped chives.

2   Cut into wedges and serve immediately.

Nutrition Info

Calories: 157kcal, Carbohydrates: 1g, Protein: 9g

DINNER

Chinese chicken salad recipe

Prep Time: 5 mins, Servings 2-4

Ingredients

For the dressing:

- 1/2 cup vegetable oil

- 1/4 cup unseasoned rice wine vinegar
- 1 tablespoon Dijon mustard
- 1 tablespoon low-sodium soy sauce
- 1 teaspoon sesame oil
- 2 garlic cloves, minced
- 1/4-inch piece of ginger, peeled and chopped
- Pinch of salt

For the salad:

- 2 cooked (grilled or roasted) chicken breasts, shredded
- 4 cups shredded green cabbage
- 1 cup shredded red cabbage
- 1 small carrot, cut into thin strips
- 1/4 cup cooked edamame
- 1/2 cup chopped cilantro leaves
- 2 tablespoons chopped mint leaves
- 4 scallions, thinly sliced
- Wonton strips (optional)

Instructions

1   Place all of the dressing ingredients in a blender, and pulse until smooth. Set aside. Combine all of the salad ingredients in a large mixing bowl. Toss with the dressing. Top with wonton strips, if desired.

Nutrition Info:

Calories 327 Calories from Fat 207, Carbohydrates 1g, Protein 30g

DAY 22

BREAKFAST

Green Shakshuka

Prep/Cook Time: 55 min, 4 servings

Ingredients

- 2 tablespoons extra-virgin olive oil
- 1 onion, minced
- 2 garlic cloves, minced
- 1 jalapeño, seeded and minced
- 1 pound spinach (thawed if frozen)
- 1 teaspoon dried cumin
- 3/4 teaspoon coriander
- Salt and freshly ground black pepper
- 2 tablespoons harissa
- 1/2 cup vegetable broth
- 8 large eggs
- Chopped fresh parsley, as needed for serving
- Chopped fresh cilantro, as needed for serving
- Red-pepper flakes, as needed for serving

Instructions

1 Preheat the oven to 350°F.
2 In a large, oven-safe skillet, heat the olive oil over medium heat. Add the onion and sauté until tender, 4 to 5 minutes. Add the garlic and jalapeño, then sauté until fragrant, 1 minute more.
3 Stir in the spinach and cook until fully wilted if using fresh, 4 to 5 minutes, or until heated through if thawed from frozen, 1 to 2 minutes.
4 Season with cumin, coriander, salt, pepper and harissa. Cook

about 1 minute, until fragrant.

5 Transfer the mixture to the bowl of a food processor or a blender and puree until coarse. Add the broth and puree until thick and smooth.

6 Wipe out the skillet and grease it with nonstick cooking spray. Pour the spinach mixture back into the pan and use a wooden spoon to make eight circular wells.

7 Gently crack the eggs into the wells. Transfer the skillet to the oven and cook until the egg whites are fully set, but the yolks are still a little bit jiggly, 20 to 25 minutes.

8 Sprinkle the shakshuka with parsley, cilantro and red-pepper flakes, to taste. Serve immediately.

Nutrition Info

251 calories, 17g fat, 10g carbs, 17g protein, 3g sugars

LUNCH

Turmeric Chickpea Cakes

Prep & Cook time: 15 minutes, Servings 4

Ingredients

- 1 small onion
- 2 cloves of garlic
- 1 can rinsed and drained chickpeas (or 1 1/2 cups pre-cooked)
- small bunch of fresh parsley, roughly chopped (about 1/4 cup)
- 2 tablespoons potato starch
- 1-2 teaspoons of sea salt freshly ground black pepper
- 1 teaspoon turmeric powder
- 1/2 – 1 teaspoon cayenne pepper (optional)
- 2 tablespoons chickpea flour + extra 3 tablespoons for coating grape seed oil for cooking

Instructions

1　In a large cast iron pan, drizzle in a little grape seed oil and fry the onion and garlic until slightly golden but not burned. Remove from heat and allow to cool.

2　In a food processor, process the chickpeas until they turn to a slightly textured paste, be sure to turn off the food processor and scrape down the sides to get all the chickpeas ground up. Add in onion and garlic, salt, pepper, turmeric and cayenne pepper and mix to fully combine. Turn the food processor off and stir in the chopped parsley.

3　(If you do have kids, I would omit the cayenne pepper entirely as most kids are not into spicy foods. Or divide the batch into two and season them differently for kiddos and adults.)

4　Take a large plate and sprinkle a few tablespoons of chickpea flour onto it. Using a spoon, scoop some of the mixture with onto your hands and shape into a ball, the size of a golf ball, and then press gently to make a patty. Drop into the chickpea flour to coat evenly. If too much flour sticks to the patty then gently dust it off with your fingers or a pastry brush. You should have a very light coating all over the patties/ burgers.

5　Reheat that same large cast iron pan to medium heat. Drizzle in a little more oil and place the patties in to cook. Cook for about 2-3 minutes on each side until the bottom is nicely browned.

6　Serve with a big salad for a healthy lunch or dinner. Or with cut up veggies on the side for kids. Makes a great party small-plates or potluck party dish!

7　Enjoy!

Nutrition Info

Calories: 268, Fat: 12.9, Sodium: 167, Protein: 33, Cholesterol: 118

DINNER

Roasted Root Veggies & Greens over Spiced Lentils

Prep/Cook Time: 45 m, 2 servings

Ingredients

- Lentils
- 1 1/2 cups water
- 1/2 cup black beluga lentils or French green lentils
- 1 teaspoon garlic powder
- 1/2 teaspoon ground coriander
- 1/2 teaspoon ground cumin
- 1/4 teaspoon ground allspice
- 1/4 teaspoon kosher salt
- 2 tablespoons lemon juice
- 1 teaspoon extra-virgin olive oil
- Vegetables
- 1 tablespoon extra-virgin olive oil
- 1 clove garlic, smashed
- 1 1/2 cups roasted root vegetables
- 2 cups chopped kale or beet greens
- 1 teaspoon ground coriander
- 1/2 teaspoon ground pepper
- Pinch of kosher salt
- 2 tablespoons tahini or low-fat plain yogurt
- Fresh parsley for garnish

Instructions

1   To prepare lentils: Combine water, lentils, garlic powder, ½ teaspoon coriander, cumin, allspice, ¼ teaspoon salt and sumac (if using) in a medium pot. Bring to a boil. Reduce heat to maintain a simmer, cover and cook until tender, 25 to 30 minutes. Uncover and continue simmering until the li q uid

reduces slightly, about 5 minutes more. Drain. Stir in lemon juice and 1 teaspoon oil. Meanwhile, to prepare vegetables: Heat oil in a large skillet over medium heat. Add garlic and cook until fragrant, 1 to 2 minutes. Add roasted root vegetables and cook, stirring often, until heated through, 2 to 4 minutes. Stir in kale (or beet greens) and cook until just wilted, 2 to 3 minutes. Stir in coriander, pepper and salt. Serve the vegetables over the lentils, topped with tahini (or yogurt). Garnish with parsley, if desired.

2   Tip: We like black beluga lentils or French green lentils instead of brown when we want lentils that hold their shape (instead of breaking down) when cooked. Look for them in natural-foods stores and some supermarkets.

Nutrition Info

453 calories; 22 g fat(3 g sat); 14 g fiber; 50 g carbohydrates; 18 g protein; 81 mcg

DAY 23

BREAKFAST

Yogurt parfait recipe with raspberries
and chia seeds

Prep/Cook Time: 20 mins, Servings 2

Ingredients

- 1/2 cup fresh raspberries
- 2 tablespoons chia seeds
- 1 teaspoon maple syrup
- Pinch of cinnamon
- 16-ounces plain yogurt
- Fresh fruit, such as sliced blackberries, nectarines, strawberries, etc.

Instructions

1   Place the raspberries in a small mixing bowl. Using the back of a fork, mash the berries until they reach a jam-like consistency. Add the chia seeds, honey, and cinnamon to the bowl. Continue to mash until all of the ingredients are fully incorporated. Set aside.

2   Place a layer of yogurt in the bottom of a medium-size glass or jar. Top with a layer of the raspberry chia mixture. Finish with an additional layer of yogurt. Garnish with fresh sliced fruit and an extra drizzle of maple syrup, if desired. Repeat with the second glass/jar.

Nutrition Info:

Calories: 264 Fat: 11 Carbohydrates: 6 Protein: 23

LUNCH

GLOW Getter Roasted Carrot
Butternut Squash Soup

Prep/Cook Time: 40, Servings 4

Ingredients

- 1 pound carrots, chopped into similar size pieces
- 1 medium (about 1 ½ pounds) butternut squash, peeled and chopped into similar size pieces
- 1/2 cup shallots, sliced
- 2 Tablespoons avocado oil
- 4 cup vegetable stock
- 1 can full-fat coconut milk
- 1 Tablespoon fresh ginger, grated*
- 1 teaspoon salt
- Freshly ground black pepper

For garnish:

- Coconut milk Cilantro
- Roasted chickpeas

Instructions

1 Preheat oven to 400 degrees.
2 Place the carrots, butternut s q uash and sliced shallots on a parchment-lined baking sheet.
3 Drizzle with avocado oil and sprinkle with salt. Lightly toss to coat.
4 Roast for 30 minutes, or until carrots and s q uash are fork tender.
5 Once cooled slightly, transfer to a blender along with the vegetable stock, coconut milk, ginger, salt and pepper. You might need to do this in two batches if you have a smaller

blender.

6   Blend until smooth and creamy, adding additional stock or water to thin if needed (you could also use a hand immersion blender for this).

7   Garnish with a drizzle of coconut milk, fresh cilantro and roasted chickpeas.

Nutrition Info

Calories 430, Calories from Fat 400, Total Fat 45g, Saturated Fat, 25g, Cholesterol 205mg, Protein 41g

----

DINNER

Roasted Salmon with Smoky Chickpeas & Greens

Prep/Cook Time 40 m, 4 servings

Ingredients

- 2 tablespoons extra-virgin olive oil, divided
- 1 tablespoon smoked paprika
- ½ teaspoon salt, divided, plus a pinch
- 1 (15 ounce) can no-salt-added chickpeas, rinsed
- 1/3 cup buttermilk
- 1/4 cup mayonnaise
- 1/4 cup chopped fresh chives and/or dill, plus more for garnish
- 1/2 teaspoon ground pepper, divided
- 1/4 teaspoon garlic powder
- 10 cups chopped kale
- 1/4 cup water
- 1 1/4 pounds wild salmon, cut into 4 portions

Instructions

1   Position racks in upper third and middle of oven; preheat to

425°F. Combine 1 tablespoon oil, paprika and 1/4 teaspoon salt in a medium bowl. Very thoroughly pat chickpeas dry, then toss with the paprika mixture.

2   Spread on a rimmed baking sheet. Bake the chickpeas on the upper rack, stirring twice, for 30 minutes. Meanwhile, puree buttermilk, mayonnaise, herbs, 1/4 teaspoon pepper and garlic powder in a blender until smooth.

3   Set aside. Heat the remaining 1 tablespoon oil in a large skillet over medium heat. Add kale and cook, stirring occasionally, for 2 minutes.

4   Add water and continue cooking until the kale is tender, about 5 minutes more. Remove from heat and stir in a pinch of salt.

5   Remove the chickpeas from the oven and push them to one side of the pan. Place salmon on the other side and season with the remaining 1/4 teaspoon each salt and pepper. Bake until the salmon is just cooked through, 5 to 8 minutes.

6   Drizzle the reserved dressing on the salmon, garnish with more herbs, if desired, and serve with the kale and chickpeas.

Nutrition Info

447 calories; 22 g fat(4 g sat); 6 g fiber; 23 g carbohydrates; 37 g protein

DAY 24

BREAKFAST

Kale Pineapple Smoothie

Prep/Cook Time: 4 mins, Servings: 1 large or 2 small smoothies

Ingredients

- 2 cups lightly packed chopped kale leaves — stems removed
- 3/4 cup unsweetened vanilla almond milk — or any milk you like
- 1 frozen medium banana — cut into chunks
- 1/4 cup plain non-fat Greek yogurt
- 1/4 cup frozen pineapple pieces
- 2 tablespoons peanut butter — creamy or crunchy (natural creamy was used)
- 1 to 3 teaspoons honey — to taste

Instructions

1 Place all ingredients (kale, almond milk, banana, yogurt, pineapple, peanut butter, and honey) in a blender in the order listed. Blend until smooth. Add more milk as needed to reach desired consistency. Enjoy immediately.

Nutrition Info

Calories: 187, Fat: 9g, Saturated Fat: 1g, Cholesterol: 3mg, Sodium: 149mg, Carbohydrates: 27g, Fiber: 4g

----

LUNCH

Kale Caesar Salad with Grilled Chicken Wrap

Prep time: 10 minute(s), Servings: 2

Ingredients

- 8 ounces grilled chicken, thinly sliced
- 6 cups curly kale, cut into bite sized pieces
- 1 cup cherry tomatoes, quartered
- 3/4 cup finely shredded Parmesan cheese
- 1/2 coddled egg (cooked about 1 minute)
- 1 clove garlic, minced
- 1/2 teaspoon Dijon mustard
- 1 teaspoon honey or agave
- 1/8 cup fresh lemon juice
- 1/8 cup olive oil
- Kosher salt and freshly ground black pepper
- 2 Lavash flat breads or two large tortillas

Instructions

1 In a bowl, mix together the half of a coddled egg, minced garlic, mustard, honey, lemon juice and olive oil. Whisk until you have formed a dressing. Season to taste with salt and pepper.

2 Add the kale, chicken and cherry tomatoes and toss to coat with the dressing and 1/4 cup of the shredded parmesan.

3 Spread out the two lavash flatbreads. Evenly distribute the salad over the two wraps and sprinkle each with 1/4 cup of parmesan.

4 Roll up the wraps and slice in half. Eat immediately

Nutrition Info:

Calories: 511, Total Fat: 37g, Saturated Fat: 13g, Trans Fat: 0g, Unsaturated Fat: 20g

----

DINNER

Almond-Matcha Green Smoothie Bowl

Prep/Cook Time 10 m, 1 serving

Ingredients

- 1/2 cup frozen sliced banana
- 1/2 cup frozen sliced peaches
- 1 cup fresh spinach
- 1/2 cup unsweetened almond milk
- 5 tablespoons slivered almonds, divided
- 1 1/2 teaspoons matcha tea powder
- 1 teaspoon maple syrup
- 1/2 ripe kiwi, diced

Instructions

1 Blend banana, peaches, spinach, almond milk, 3 tablespoons almonds, matcha and maple syrup in a blender until very smooth. Pour the smoothie into a bowl and top with kiwi and the remaining 2 tablespoons slivered almonds.

Nutrition info

353 calories; 19 g fat(1 g sat); 9 g fiber; 44 g carbohydrates; 10 g protein; 70 mcg

☆☆☆☆☆

DAY 25

BREAKFAST

Mushroom and Spinach Frittata

Prep/Cook Time: 45 MIN, Servings 4

Ingredients

- 6 eggs
- 1/4 cup (60 ml) milk
- 1 cup (250 ml) grated cheddar cheese
- 1 onion, thinly sliced
- 4 oz (115 g) white button mushrooms, sliced
- 3 tablespoons (45 ml) butter
- 2 cups (500 ml) baby spinach,
- Salt and pepper

Instructions

1 With the rack in the middle position, preheat the oven to 180 °C (350 °F). Butter a 20- cm (8-inch) square baking dish. Set aside.

2 In a large bowl, combine eggs and milk with a whisk. Add cheese. Season with salt and pepper. Place bowl aside.

3 In a large non-stick skillet, brown onion and mushrooms in butter over medium heat. Season with salt and pepper. Add spinach and continue cooking for about 1 minute, stirring constantly.

4 Pour mushroom mixture into egg mixture. Stir well and pour into baking dish. Bake the frittata for about 25 minutes or until lightly browned and puffed. Cut frittata into four s q uares and remove from dish with a spatula. Place on a plate and voila, it is ready to serve warm or cold.

Nutrition Info: Calories:

240kcal, Carbohydrates: 1g, Protein: 24g, Fat: 15g

LUNCH

Buddha Bowl with Kale, Avocado, Orange and Wild Rice

Prep/Cook Time: 40 min, 2 servings

Ingredients

Rice

- 1 cup wild rice
- 3 cups vegetable broth or water
- 1 garlic clove, minced
- 2 tablespoons extra-virgin olive oil
- 2 tablespoons rice vinegar
- 1 tablespoon chopped fresh mint
- Salt and freshly ground black pepper

Toppings

- 1 bunch kale, roughly chopped
- 2 tablespoons olive oil
- 1 tablespoon rice vinegar
- 1/4 cup pomegranate seeds
- 1 orange, cut into segments
- 1/2 avocado, sliced
- 1/4 cup pumpkin seeds
- 2 hard-boiled eggs
- Salt and freshly ground black pepper

Instructions

1 Make the Rice: In a medium pot, stir the rice with the broth

(or water, if using) and garlic to combine. Bring the mixture to a simmer over medium-high heat.

2   Once the li q uid is boiling, reduce the heat to low and simmer until the rice is tender and all the li q uid has been absorbed, 15 to 17 minutes.

3   Let the rice cool for 5 to 10 minutes and then toss it with the olive oil, vinegar, mint, salt and pepper.

4   Make the Toppings: In a medium bowl, toss the kale with the olive oil and vinegar. Divide the rice between two bowls and then top with e q ual amounts of kale.

5   Top each of the bowls with 2 tablespoons pomegranate seeds, half the orange slices, half the avocado slices, 2 tablespoons pumpkin seeds and a hard-boiled egg. Season the egg with salt and pepper. Serve immediately.

Nutrition Info

417 calories, 15g fat, 62g carbs, 12g protein, 2g sugars

DINNER

Easy Saag Paneer

Prep/Cook Time 25 m, 4 servings

Ingredients

- 8 ounces paneer cheese, cut into 1/2-inch cubes
- 1/4 teaspoon ground turmeric
- 2 tablespoons extra-virgin olive oil, divided
- 1 small onion, finely chopped
- 1 jalapeño pepper, finely chopped (optional)
- 1 clove garlic, minced
- 1 tablespoon minced fresh ginger
- 2 teaspoons garam masala

- 1 teaspoon ground cumin
- 20 ounces frozen spinach, thawed and finely chopped
- 3/4 teaspoon salt
- 2 cups low-fat plain yogurt

Instructions

1   Toss paneer with turmeric in a medium bowl until coated. Heat 1 tablespoon oil in a large nonstick skillet over medium heat. Add the paneer and cook, flipping once, until browned on both sides, about 5 minutes. Transfer to a plate. Add the remaining 1 tablespoon oil to the pan.

2   Add onion and jalapeño (if using) and cook, stirring frequently, until golden brown, 7 to 8 minutes. (If the pan seems dry during cooking, add a little water, 2 tablespoons at a time.) Add garlic, ginger, garam masala and cumin.

3   Cook, stirring, until fragrant, about 30 seconds. Add spinach and salt. Cook, stirring, until hot, about 3 minutes. Remove from the heat and stir in yogurt and paneer.

Nutrition Info

382 calories, 24 g fat(12 g sat), 5 g fiber, 19 g carbohydrates, 25 g protein, 223 mcg folate, 64 mg cholesterol

DAY 26

BREAKFAST

Overnight Oats with Blueberries
and Almonds

Prep/Cook Time: 8 hr 5 min, 1 serving

Ingredients

Oats

- 3/4 cup old-fashioned oats
- 1/2 to 3/4 cup milk (such as whole, skim, almond, soy or coconut)
- 1 tablespoon maple syrup

Toppings

- 1/3 cup yogurt
- 3 tablespoons sliced almonds
- 1/4 cup blueberries

Instructions

1. Make the Oats: Pour the oats into a 1-pint mason jar.
2. In a small bowl, mix the milk with the maple syrup. (If you prefer a thicker oatmeal, use less milk.)
3. Pour the milk mixture into the jar. Screw on the lid and refrigerate overnight, about 8 hours.
4. Make the Toppings: In the morning, top the oatmeal with the yogurt, sliced almonds and blueberries. Eat immediately or screw the top on and take it on the go.

Nutrition Info:

367 calories, 9g fat, 62g carbs, 13g protein, 21g sugars

LUNCH

Healing Carrot Soup with Turmeric and Ginger

Prep/Cook Time: 20 mins, Servings 2

Ingredients

- 4 carrots, peeled and chopped
- 1 parsnip, peeled and chopped
- 1 yellow onion, roughly chopped
- 4 garlic cloves, crushed
- 2 teaspoons virgin coconut oil
- 3 cups low sodium vegetable broth, warm
- 1 teaspoon turmeric powder
- 1-inch ginger knob, peeled and grated
- Juice from 1/2 of a lemon
- Pinch cayenne pepper
- Fresh parsley, Greek yogurt, black sesame, coconut flakes, to serve

Instructions

1 Preheat the oven to 350°F.
2 Line a baking sheet with parchment paper. Add the carrots, parsnip, onion and garlic, then season with turmeric and cayenne, drizzle with coconut oil and toss to coat evenly. Roast for 15 minutes, then remove from the oven and transfer into a blender with the vegetable broth, lemon juice and ginger.
3 Blend the ingredients until smooth and creamy.
4 Pour the soup into serving bowls, garnish with fresh parsley, sesame and coconut flakes, drizzle with Greek yogurt and serve warm.

Nutrition Info

Calories: 323kcal, Carbohydrates: 21g, Protein: 50g, Fat: 16g

----

DINNER

Polenta with Wild Mushroom Bolognese

Servings 4

Ingredients

For the polenta:

- 6 cups vegetable stock
- 2 cups yellow cornmeal
- 2 tablespoons unsalted butter
- 1/4 cup grated Parmesan cheese

For the wild mushroom Bolognese:

- 1 onion, chopped
- 2 carrots, peeled and chopped
- 2 celery stalks, peeled and chopped
- 2 garlic cloves, chopped
- 1/4 cup olive oil
- 1/2 teaspoon dried thyme
- 1 teaspoon dried oregano
- 6-ounces assorted wild mushrooms (if you can't find wild mushrooms, you can substitute for a mix of Cremini and White Button varieties.)
- 1 teaspoon salt
- 1/2 teaspoon black pepper
- 1/2 cup red wine
- 1 28-ounce can chopped tomatoes

Instructions

1 To make the polenta (you can do this before you make the Bolognese, or while the Bolognese is simmering.): Bring the

stock to a boil.

2   Slowly whisk in the cornmeal, removing any lumps as you go.

3   Reduce the heat to medium-low, and allow the cornmeal to cook for approximately 15- 20 minutes, until thickened. It should have a similar consistency to porridge.

4   Remove the polenta from the heat, and stir in the butter and Parmesan cheese. Set aside. To make the Bolognese: Place the onion, carrots, celery, and garlic in a food processor and pulse until the vegetables are finely chopped – but not pureed. Set aside.

5   Heat the olive oil over medium heat, in a large pot. Add the chopped vegetables to the pot. Cook for approximately 5 minutes, just until tender.

6   Add the spices and mushrooms to the pan. Cook for an additional 5 minutes, until all of the water has evaporated from the mushrooms.

7   Pour in the red wine, scraping up any brown bits that have accumulated at the bottom of the pan.

8   Add the tomatoes to the mixture and bring to a boil. Reduce the heat to medium-low and continue to simmer for an additional 15 minutes.

9   Serve the sauce atop the polenta.

Nutrition Info

Calories: 420kcal, Carbohydrates: 23g, Protein: 30g

DAY 27

BREAKFAST

Chia Quinoa Porridge

Prep/Cook Time: 7 mins, Servings: 2

Ingredients

- 1 cup thick cashew milk
- 2 cups cooked quinoa
- 1 cup fresh organic blueberries (or frozen)
- 1/4 cup toasted walnuts
- 1/2 tsp ground cinnamon
- 2 tsp raw honey
- 1 Tbsp chia seeds

Instructions

1 Combine the quinoa and cashew milk in a saucepan and slowly warm over medium low heat.
2 Stir in blueberries, cinnamon and walnuts until all are evenly warmed. Remove from heat and stir in raw honey. Top with chia seeds.
3 Serve in bowls and top with raw cacao nibs for an added pop of antioxidants.

Nutrition Info

Calories 340 Calories from Fat 342, Saturated Fat 15g, Sodium 809mg, Potassium 712mg, Carbohydrates 6.5g

----

LUNCH

Grilled Salmon & Butter Lettuce Taco Wraps with Avocado Sauce Recipe

Prep/Cook Time: 15 mins, Servingss: 4-6 salmon

Ingredients

- 1-2 tbsp Everyday Seasoning Salt recipe link here (or substitute with your favorite grilled fish seasoning)
- 1/4 cup Avocado Sauce recipe link here
- 2 fresh salmon fish fillets
- 1 head of butter lettuce (aka Boston or bibb lettuce)
- 2-3 cup cole slaw mix or shredded cabbage
- 1/4 cup fresh cilantro leaves, chopped
- 1 lime, juiced
- Salt, to taste

Instructions

1   Ideally, prepare the Everyday Seasoning Salt and Avocado Sauce before starting
2   Season salmon filets generously with Everyday Seasoning Salt (or your favorite seasoning). Lightly pat to adhere, and drizzle with some olive oil or avocado oil
3   Heat grill to medium high. Grill salmon 5-8 minutes, turning once. Cook just until fillets easily flake but are still moist. Remove from grill and set aside temporarily to cool. (Instead of grilling, salmon fillets can be pan-fried or baked if desired)
4   In a small mixing bowl, combine cole slaw mix (or shredded cabbage) with chopped cilantro leaves and juice of 1 lime. Salt to taste
5   Rinse butter lettuce leaves, and spin-dry in salad spinner, or lightly blot dry with paper towels. Select the best cup- shaped leaves to create your lettuce wrap tacos

6   Break apart cooled salmon fillets. Place salmon pieces inside lettuce wrap tacos, and sprinkle each with cole slaw mixture

7   Finish each lettuce wrap taco with a healthy drizzle of Avocado Sauce

Nutrition Info

Calories: 364kcal, Carbohydrates: 2.2g, Protein: 30g, Fat: 37g, Saturated Fat: 14g

----

DINNER

Gut-Healing Salmon & Cauliflower Rice Bowl

Prep/Cook Time: 1 hr 10 mins, Servings 2

Ingredients

- 2 salmon fillets, sustainably sourced or organic
- 10 to 12 Brussels sprouts, chopped in half
- 1 bunch kale, washed and shredded
- 1/2 head cauliflower, pulsed into cauliflower rice (you can use a whole cauliflower head if you wish)
- 3 tablespoons olive or coconut oil
- 1 teaspoon curry powder Himalayan salt

For marinade

- 1/4 cup tamari sauce
- 1 teaspoon Dijon mustard
- 1 teaspoon sesame oil
- 1 teaspoon honey or maple syrup (optional)
- 1 tablespoon sesame seeds

Instructions

1   Preheat oven to 350°F.

2   Line a baking tray and add chopped Brussels sprouts. Coat

with 1 tablespoon oil and season with salt. Add to oven and roast for 20 minutes.

3   Meanwhile, make marinade by combining all ingredients in a bowl and whisking until combined.

4   Remove Brussels sprouts after 20 minutes and add salmon fillets to the baking tray. Spoon marinade over salmon fillets and return to oven for a further 13 to 15 minutes, or until salmon is cooked to your liking.

5   While salmon is cooking, heat a pan over medium-high heat and add 1 tablespoon oil. Add kale and sauté until wilted (2 to 3 minutes). Remove from pan and set aside.

6   Heat remaining oil in pan and add cauliflower rice. Season with 1 teaspoon curry powder and salt and sauté until cooked (2 to 3 minutes).

7   Remove salmon and Brussels sprouts from oven and divide into two bowls. Add sautéed kale and cauliflower rice to bowls.

Nutrition Info

Calories 234 kcal, Net carbs7.6 grams, Protein37.3 grams

DAY 28

BREAKFAST

Buckwheat Cinnamon & Ginger Granola

Prep/Cook Time: 50 mins, Servings 2-4

Ingredients:

- 2 cups of gluten-free oats
- 1 cup of buckwheat groats
- 1 cup of sunflower seeds
- 1/2 cup of pumpkin seeds
- 1/4 cup Chia seeds
- 1/2 Cup Coconut Flakes
- 1 1/2 Cup mixed Raw nuts – I love almonds, pecans, hazelnuts and walnuts
- 4 tbsp of coconut oil
- 1 tsp Ground Cinnamon
- 1 1/2 - 2inch piece of ginger
- 2 tbsp nut butter
- 1/3 cup or Rice Malt Syrup or Raw Honey
- 4 tbsp of raw cacao powder – Optional

Instructions:

1 Pre-heat the oven to 180C
2 Place the nuts into your food processer and quickly blitz to roughly chop (I love to keep the chopped pieces quite large for that extra crunch!)
3 Place the chopped nuts into a large mixing bowl and add all other dry ingredients mixing well to combine – oats, buckwheat, seeds, coconut, cinnamon and salt
4 In a saucepan over a low heat gently melt the coconut oil, nut butter and honey/rice malt syrup together

5   Peel and grate the ginger and mix into the wet mixture.

6   Add the cacao powder (if using) to the wet mixture and combine well

7   Pour the wet mixture over the dry mixture and mix well making sure everything is coated

8   Transfer the mixture into a large baking tray lined with grease-proof paper or greased with coconut oil. Be sure to spread the mixture out evenly

9   Bake for 35-40 mins, turning the mixture halfway. Bake until the granola is golden and crispy!

10 Allow for the granola to cool before placing it in an airtight container and store for up to 2 weeks.

11 Serve with your favourite nut milk, a scoop of coconut yoghurt, fresh fruit and your favourite superfoods – goji berries, flax seeds, bee pollen….whatever you fancy! Mix it up daily.

Nutrition Info

Calories: 354, Saturated Fat 5.6g, Cholesterol 149.7mg, Total Carbohydrate 6.7g, Sugars 1.8g, Protein 45.4g

----

LUNCH

Golden Sun-Dried Tomato Red Lentil Pasta.

Prep/Cook Time 40 minutes, Servings 6 servings

Ingredients

- 1/4 cup extra virgin olive oil
- 1 sweet onion, chopped
- 6 cloves garlic, minced or grated
- 1 tablespoon dried basil

- 1 tablespoon dried oregano
- 2 teaspoons ground turmeric kosher salt and pepper
- 1 (28 ounce) can fire roasted tomatoes, I like san marzano
- 1/2 cup oil packed sun-dried tomatoes, oil drained + chopped
- 1 tablespoon apple cider vinegar
- 1 (8 ounce) box red lentil pasta or other short cut pasta
- 2 large handfuls baby spinach or kale
- grated parmesan, nutritional yeast, toasted pine nuts and or seeds, for topping

Instructions

1   Heat the olive oil in a large pot over medium heat. When the oil shimmers, add the onion and cook until soft and caramelized, about 5-10 minutes. Add the garlic, basil, oregano, turmeric, salt and pepper. Cook for 1 minute or until fragrant. Slowly add the tomatoes and the juices from the can, crushing the tomatoes with the back of a wooden spoon. Add the sun-dried tomatoes and vinegar. Simmer the sauce for 10-15 minutes or until reduced slightly. If desired, you can puree the sauce in a blender.

2   Stir in the spinach and cook five minutes longer.

3   Meanwhile, bring a large pot of salted water to a boil and boil the pasta to al dente according to package Instructions. Drain.

4   Divide the pasta among bowls and top with a generous amount of sauce. Top as desired with cheese, nuts and herbs.

Nutrition Info

Calories: 231kcal, Carbohydrates: 3g, Sodium: 474mg, Potassium: 110mg, Fiber: 0.01g, Sugar: 1g

----

DINNER

Lentil and Chicken Soup with
Sweet Potatoes and Escarole

Prep/Cook Time 35 minutes, 4–6 servings

Ingredients

- 1 cooked chicken carcass (from 1 store-bought rotisserie chicken or homemade roast chicken)
- 1 lb. sweet potatoes (about 2 medium), peeled, cut into 1" pieces
- 3/4 cup French lentils (about 5 oz.), rinsed
- 1 tsp. kosher salt, plus more
- 2 Tbsp. extra-virgin olive oil
- 10 celery stalks, sliced on the bias into 1/4" slices
- 6 garlic cloves, thinly sliced
- 1 1/2 cups shredded cooked chicken (from 1/2 of a store-bought rotisserie chicken or homemade roast chicken)
- 1/2 head escarole, cut into bite-size pieces
- 1/2 cup finely chopped dill
- 2 Tbsp. fresh lemon juice

Instructions

1 Place chicken carcass, potatoes, lentils, and 1 tsp. salt in a large pot. Cover with 8 cups water. Bring to a boil over high heat, skimming off any foam, then reduce heat to medium-low and simmer until potatoes are fork tender and lentils are cooked through, 10–12 minutes. Discard chicken carcass.

2 Meanwhile, heat oil in a large heavy skillet over medium-high. Add celery and garlic and cook, stirring often, until celery and garlic are lightly golden brown and tender, about 12 minutes.

3 Stir celery, garlic, shredded chicken, and escarole into soup

and cook, stirring occasionally, until escarole is wilted, about 5 minutes. Remove from heat. Stir in dill and lemon juice; season soup with salt.

Nutrition Info

Calories 529, Carbohydrates 34 g, Fat 31 g, Protein 28 g, Saturated Fat 8 g, Sodium 491 mg

DAY 29

BREAKFAST

Amaranth Porridge with Roasted Pears

Prep/Cook Time: 40 mins, Servings: 2 servings

Ingredients

Porridge

- 1/2 cup uncooked amaranth
- 1/2 cup water
- 1 cup 2% milk
- 1/4 teaspoon salt Pears
- 1 teaspoon maple syrup
- 1 large pear
- 1/2 teaspoon ground cinnamon
- 1/4 teaspoon ground ginger
- 1/8 teaspoon ground nutmeg
- 1/8 teaspoon ground clove

Pecan/Pear Topping

- 2 tablespoons pecan pieces
- 1 teaspoon pure maple syrup
- 1 cup plain 0% Greek yogurt, for serving

Instructions

1   Preheat oven to 400°.

2   Drain and rinse amaranth. Combine with one cup milk, water, and salt. Bring amaranth to a boil, and reduce to a simmer (all the way to low.) Cover and let simmer for 25 minutes until the amaranth is soft but there is still some li q uid left. Remove from heat and let sit for 5 to 10 more minutes to thicken amaranth. Add a bit more milk to thin the texture out if

desired.

3   Toss together the 1 teaspoon maple syrup with the pecan pieces. Roast until the pecans are toasted and the maple syrup has dried, 10 to 15 minutes. Pecans will become q uite fragrant when done. Pecans will crisp as they cool.

4   Along with the pecans, dice the pears and toss with the remaining 1 teaspoon of maple syrup and spices. Roast in a roasting pan for 15 minutes, until the pears are tender.

5   Stir in 3/4 of the roasted pears in the porridge. Divide yogurt into two bowls and top with porridge, roasted pecans, and the remaining pear pieces.

Nutrition Info

Calories: 510kcal, Carbohydrates: 8g, Protein: 53g, Fat: 39g, Saturated Fat: 16g

----

LUNCH

Quick and Easy Quinoa Orange Salad

Prep Time: 10 mins, Servings 1

Ingredients

- 1 cup cooked quinoa, cooled
- 2 small oranges, supremed
- 1 celery rib, finely chopped
- 20g Brazil nuts, chopped
- 1 green onion, sliced
- 1/4 cup fresh parsley, finely chopped

For the dressing

- juice from above oranges
- 1/2 tsp lemon juice

- 1/2 tsp fresh ginger, grated
- 1 tsp white wine vinegar
- 1 small clove garlic, minced
- 1/2 tsp salt
- 1/4 tsp black pepper pinch cinnamon

Instructions

1. Cut the oranges into supremes, working over a bowl, in order not lose any of the juice. When you've got all your supremes done, make sure to s q ueeze all the juice out of the "membranes" that are left behind.

2. Transfer that juice to your mini blender or food processor. Add the rest of the ingredients for the dressing and blend until smooth.

3. Cut your orange supremes into bite size pieces and add them to a medium size mixing bowl. Add the rest of the ingredients, including the dressing, and stir until well combined.

4. Serve immediately, or keep in the refrigerator until ready to serve.

Nutrition Info

Calories: 223, Total Fat: 30.9g, Carbohydrates: 7.4g, Dietary Fiber: 1.6g, Protein: 44g

----

DINNER

Baked Tilapia Recipe with Pecan
Rosemary Topping

Prep/Cook Time 33 mins, Servings 4

Ingredients

- 1/3 cup chopped raw pecans
- 1/3 cup whole wheat panko breadcrumbs

- 2 tsp chopped fresh rosemary
- 1/2 tsp coconut palm sugar or brown sugar
- 1/8 tsp salt
- 1 pinch cayenne pepper
- 1 1/2 tsp olive oil
- 1 egg white
- 4 (4 oz. each) tilapia fillets

Instructions

1. Preheat oven to 350 degrees F.
2. In a small baking dish, stir together pecans, breadcrumbs, rosemary, coconut palm sugar, salt and cayenne pepper. Add the olive oil and toss to coat the pecan mixture.
3. Bake until the pecan mixture is light golden brown, 7 to 8 minutes.
4. Increase the heat to 400 degrees F. Coat a large glass baking dish with cooking spray.
5. In a shallow dish, whisk the egg white. Working with one tilapia at a time, dip the fish in the egg white and then the pecan mixture, lightly coating each side. Place the fillets in the prepared baking dish.
6. Press the remaining pecan mixture into the top of the tilapia fillets. Bake until the tilapia is just cooked through, about 10 minutes. Serve.

Nutrition Info

Calories 222.4 cal, Calories from fat 90, Total Fat 10.8g, Saturated Fat 1.4g, Cholesterol 55.0mg, Sodium 153.3mg

DAY 30

BREAKFAST

Turkey Apple Breakfast Hash

Prep/Cook Time: 20 mins, Servings: 5

Ingredients

For the meat:

- 1 lb ground turkey
- 1 tablespoon coconut oil
- 1/2 teaspoon dried thyme
- 1/2 teaspoon cinnamon
- sea salt, to taste

For the hash:

- 1 tablespoon coconut oil
- 1 onion
- large or 2 small zucchini
- 1/2 cup shredded carrots
- 2 cups cubed frozen butternut squash (or sweet potato)
- 1 large apple, peeled, cored, and chopped
- 2 cups spinach or greens of choice
- 1 teaspoon cinnamon
- 3/4 teaspoon powdered ginger
- 1/2 teaspoon garlic powder
- 1/2 teaspoon turmeric
- 1/2 teaspoon dried thyme
- sea salt, to taste

Instructions

1   Heat a tablespoon of coconut oil in a skillet over medium/high heat. Add ground turkey and cook until browned. Season with

cinnamon, thyme, and a pinch of sea salt. Move to plate.

2   Drop remaining coconut oil to the same skillet and sauté onion for 2-3 minutes, until softened.

3   Add in zucchini, carrots, apple, and frozen s q uash. Cook for 4-5 minutes, or until veggies have softened.

4   Add in spinach and stir until wilted.

5   Stir in cooked turkey, seasonings, and salt and turn off heat.

6   Enjoy this hash fresh from the skillet or let cool and refrigerate to eat throughout the week. The hash will keep for about 5-6 days in a sealed container in the refrigerator.

Nutrition Info

Calories: 342, Fat: 199, Carbohydrates: 7g, Fiber: 1g, Protein: 24g

----

LUNCH

Lettuce Wraps with Smoked Trout

Prep/Cook Time: 50 mins, Servings 4

Ingredients

- 2 medium carrots, peeled
- 1/2 unpeeled English hothouse cucumber (do not remove seeds)
- 1/4 cup thinly sliced shallots
- 1/4 cup thinly sliced jalapeño chiles with seeds (preferably red; about 2 large)
- 2 tablespoons fresh lime juice or unseasoned rice vinegar
- 1 tablespoon sugar
- 1 tablespoon fish sauce (such as nam pla or nuoc nam)*
- 2 4.5-ounce packages skinless smoked trout fillets,** broken into bite-size pieces (about 2 cups)
- 1 cup diced grape tomatoes

- 1/2 cup whole fresh mint leaves
- 1/2 cup small whole fresh basil leaves
- 16 small to medium inner leaves of romaine lettuce (from about 2 hearts of romaine)
- 1/3 cup (about) Asian sweet chili sauce***
- 1/4 cup finely chopped lightly salted dry-roasted peanuts

Instructions

1   Using vegetable peeler, shave carrots and cucumber lengthwise into ribbons. Cut ribbons into 3-inch-long sections, then cut sections into matchstick-size strips. Place in large bowl. Add shallots, jalapeños, lime juice, sugar, and fish sauce; let marinate 30 minutes at room temperature.

2   Add trout pieces and tomatoes to vegetable mixture and toss to blend. Transfer trout-vegetable mixture to large strainer and drain off li q uid. Return trout-vegetable mixture to same bowl; add mint and basil and toss to blend.

3   Arrange lettuce leaves on large platter. Divide trout-vegetable salad among lettuce leaves. Drizzle sweet chili sauce over each salad and sprinkle with peanuts.

Nutrition Info

Calories 423, Carbohydrates 60 g, Fat12 g, Protein 33 g, Saturated Fat 2 g, Sodium 1245 mg

----

DINNER

Homemade Vegetarian Chili

Prep/Cook Time: 1 hour, 4 to 6 servings

Ingredients

- 2 tablespoons extra-virgin olive oil
- 1 medium red onion, chopped

- 1 large red bell pepper, chopped
- 2 medium carrots, chopped
- 2 ribs celery, chopped
- 1 1/2 teaspoon salt, divided
- 4 cloves garlic, pressed or minced
- 2 tablespoons chili powder*
- 2 teaspoons ground cumin
- 1 1/2 teaspoons smoked paprika*
- 1 teaspoon dried oregano
- large can (28 ounces) or 2 small cans (15 ounces each) diced tomatoes**, with their juices
- 2 cans (15 ounces each) black beans, rinsed and drained
- 1 can (15 ounces) pinto beans, rinsed and drained
- 2 cups vegetable broth or water
- 1 bay leaf
- 2 tablespoons chopped fresh cilantro, plus more for garnishing
- 1 to 2 teaspoons sherry vinegar or red wine vinegar or lime juice, to taste

Garnishes:

- chopped cilantro, sliced avocado, tortilla chips, sour cream or crème fraîche, grated cheddar cheese, etc.

Instructions

1   In a large Dutch oven or heavy-bottomed pot over medium heat, warm the olive oil until shimmering. Add the chopped onion, bell pepper, carrot, celery and ¼ teaspoon of the salt. Stir to combine and cook, stirring occasionally, until the vegetables are tender and the onion is translucent, about 7 to 10 minutes.

2   Add the garlic, chili powder, cumin, smoked paprika and oregano. Cook until fragrant while stirring constantly, about 1 minute.

3   Add the diced tomatoes and their juices, the drained black beans and pinto beans, vegetable broth and bay leaf. Stir to combine and let the mixture come to a simmer. Continue cooking, stirring occasionally and reducing heat as necessary to maintain a gentle simmer, for 30 minutes. Remove the chili from the heat.

4   For the best texture and flavor, transfer 1 ½ cups of the chili to a blender, making sure to get some of the liquid portion. Securely fasten the lid and blend until smooth (watch out for hot steam), then pour the blended mixture back into the pot. (Or, you can blend the chili briefly with an immersion blender, or mash the chili with a potato masher until it reaches a thicker, more chili-like consistency.)

5   Add the chopped cilantro, stir to blend, and then mix in the vinegar, to taste. Add salt to taste, too—I added ¼ teaspoon more at this point. Divide the mixture into individual bowls and serve with garnishes of your choice. This chili will keep well in the refrigerator for about 4 days or you can freeze it for longer-term storage.

Nutrition Info:

Calories 372, Fat 25.93g, Carbohydrates 1.48g, Fiber 0.02g, Protein 28.21g

More Anti-Inflammatory Diet Recipes

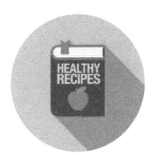

1 gluten free crepes

Prep/Cook Time: 45 mins, Servings: 10 crepes

Ingredients

Option 1.

- Make crepes using gluten-free and gum-free waffle and pancake mix 1 cup cold water
- 2 eggs
- 2 tablespoons butter , melted
- 3 tablespoons sugar
- 1/2 cups gluten-free pancake mix

Option 2.

- Make crepes using your favorite gluten-free and gum-free flour blend: 1 cup cold water
- 2 tablespoons cold water
- 2 eggs
- 2 tablespoons butter, melted
- 3 tablespoons sugar
- 1 1/2 cups gluten-free flour (gum-free multi-purpose flour such as King Arthur brand)
- 1/2 teaspoon gluten free baking powder or mix baking soda and cream of tartar in equal parts
- 1/2 teaspoon vanilla extract

Instructions

1 Mix all crepe ingredients in a large bowl and whisk the mixture until lumps dissolve. Let the mixture sit for about 15 minutes at room temperature. It will thicken after 15 minutes.

2 Heat frying pan until very hot (on high heat on stove top), spray it with oil spray (or add melted butter) and, using a soup ladle or 1/4 measuring cup, pour small amount of batter into

the frying pan as you roll the pan from side to side just enough to cover the bottom of the pan evenly with a thin layer of crepe batter. Depending on the size of your soup ladle, you could use a whole ladle-ful, or less. It also depends on the diameter of your skillet. The key is to cover the bottom of the pan with just a slightly thick layer of batter, don't coat it too thickly.

3   Let this thin layer of crepe batter cook for 1,2 or 3 minutes, depending on your pan (the subse q uent crepes will re q uire much less time to cook than the first time as the pan heats up even more), then flip the crepe to the other side and let it cook for another minute on the other side. This way, you cook each crepe 1-2 minutes on each side. To flip the crepe, pick up the sides of the crepe around its circumference, gradually reaching towards the center of the crepe from all sides, until the crepe separates from the pan. How to know when it's time to flip the crepe? When you pour the batter, it will be wet in the frying pan but gradually bubbles will be forming and batter will start to dry. When it's all bubbles and no li q uid batter – it's time to flip!

4   There is no need to spray your pan with cooking spray or grease it with butter each time, only do it once, for the first crepe. If you're using a good stainless steel pan (I use All-Clad) or non-stick pan - spraying the pan once before the first crepe is enough.

5   Your subsequent crepes might require much less time to cook, and the more of them you have to make, the faster you will have to flip the crepes, because the frying pan will get more and more heated up. When you cook crepes, your frying pan is always on high heat. This will minimize sticking.

6   As each crepe gets done, transfer it to the plate and add each new crepe on top of previous crepe in the stack. Sometimes I like to brush each crepe with softened butter and then top it with the next one (but it's not necessary). Deliciousness!

Nutrition Info

Calories 248 Calories from Fat 315, Fat 35g, Saturated Fat 13g, Potassium 589mg, Carbohydrates 3g, Protein 30g

Anti-Inflammatory Salad

Prep Time: 5 mins, Servings 4-6

Ingredients

- 24-28 oz bag Sweet Kale Salad Mix and nut/seed and dried fruit packet included*
- 1 1/2 c fresh blueberries
- 16 oz cooked, cooled, and peeled beets quartered or chopped

Turmeric Dressing

- 1/3 c extra virgin olive oil
- 2 TBSP apple cider vinegar
- 1 TBSP lemon juice
- 1 tsp turmeric
- 1 clove garlic, grated
- 1 tsp fresh grated ginger
- 1/2 sea salt
- 1/4 tsp freshly ground black pepper
- 1/2 tsp sea salt
- 1/4 tsp freshly ground black pepper

Instructions

- Mix or shake together dressing ingredients. You can also blend them together if you want a smooth dressing.
- Divide salad mix between bowls, top with beets, blueberries,

and the nut/seed mixture. Serve or drizzle with dressing.

- Enjoy!

Recipe Notes

You will use the included nut/seed and dried fruit packet that comes with the salad but not the dressing packet.

Herb-Baked Eggs

Prep/Cook Time: 5 mins, Servings 1

Ingredients

- 1 teaspoon melted butter
- 1 tablespoon milk
- 2 eggs
- Sprinkle of garlic powder, dried thyme, dried oregano, dried parsley, and dried dill

Instructions

1   Set your oven to "Broil" mode, on low.
2   Coat the bottom of a small baking dish with the butter and milk.
3   Crack the eggs on top of butter and milk combination (or crack in a separate bowl, and pour on top). Sprinkle with garlic and dried herbs.
4   Bake for 5-6 minutes, until the eggs are cooked to your liking.

Nutrition Info

Calories 318, Calories from Fat 171, Fat 19g, Carbohydrates 8g, Fiber 1g, Sugar 4g, Protein 29g

Pecan Banana Bread Overnight Oats Recipe

Prep/Cook Time: 6 hours 15 minutes, Servings 2

Ingredients

- 1 cup old-fashioned rolled oats
- 1 1/2 cups milk
- 2 very ripe bananas, mashed
- 1/4 cup plain Greek yogurt
- 2 Tbsp. unsweetened coconut flakes, toasted
- 2 Tbsp. honey
- 1 Tbsp. chia seeds
- 2 tsp. vanilla extract
- 1/4 tsp. flaked sea salt
- Banana slices, roasted pecans, fig halves, honey and pomegranate seeds, for serving

Instructions

1   In a medium bowl, stir together the oats; milk; bananas; Greek yogurt; unsweetened coconut flakes; honey; chia seeds; vanilla extract and sea salt until well combined. Divide mixture between 2 bowls or glass jars. Cover and refrigerate at least 6 hours or overnight. Stir, heat up if desired, and top with banana slices, roasted pecans and fig halves. Drizzle with honey and sprinkle with pomegranate seeds.

Nutrition Info:

Calories: 518 Fat: 40g Carbohydrates: 2g Fiber: 0g Protein: 34g

☆☆☆☆☆

Gingerbread Oatmeal Recipe

Prep/Cook Time: 35 mins, Servings: 4 servings

Ingredients

- 4 cups water
- 1 cup steel cut oats
- 1 1/2 tbsp. ground cinnamon
- 1/4 tsp. ground coriander
- 1/4 tsp. ground cloves
- 1/4 tsp. ground ginger
- 1/4 tsp. ground allspice
- 1/8 tsp. ground nutmeg
- 1/4 tsp. ground cardamom maple syrup to taste

Instructions

2   Cook the oats to package Instructions but include the spices when you add the oats to the water.

3   When finished cooking, add maple syrup to taste.

Recipe Notes

Please note that the nutrition data below is a ballpark figure. Exact data is not possible. Data below does not include maple syrup.

Nutrition Info

Calories 175, Calories from Fat 27, Total Fat 3g, Sodium 17mg

Maple-Baked Rice Porridge Recipe With Fruit

Prep/Cook Time: 40 mins, Servings 2

Ingredients

- 1/2 cup brown rice
- 1/2 teaspoon pure vanilla extract
- Pinch of cinnamon
- 2 tablespoons pure maple syrup
- Sliced fruit, such as berries, pears, plums, or cherries
- Pinch of salt (optional)

Instructions

1   Preheat the oven to 400 degrees.

2   Place the rice and 1 cup of water in a pot set over medium-high heat. Bring to a boil and add the vanilla extract and cinnamon, and stir. Cover and reduce the heat to medium-low. Simmer for approximately 10-15 minutes (or to package Instructions if you are using a variety of rice that takes longer to cook), until tender.

3   Give the rice a stir and portion it out into two heat-safe bowls. Top each bowl with a tablespoon of maple syrup and the sliced fruit of your choice. Sprinkle with salt, if desired.

4   Bake for approximately 10-15 minutes until the maple syrup is bubbling and the fruit is beginning to caramelize. Serve immediately.

Nutrition Info:

Calories 232, Total Fat 16g, Saturated Fat 5g, Cholesterol 98mg, Sodium 844mg Fiber 1g, Sugar 2g, Protein 20g

Buckwheat Berry Pancakes

Prep/Cook Time: 20 min, Servings: 4 servings

Ingredients

- 3/4 cup buckwheat flour
- 3/4 cup whole-wheat pastry flour
- 1 1/2 teaspoons baking powder
- 1/2 teaspoon baking soda
- 1/4 teaspoon salt
- 1 cup buttermilk
- 3/4 cup nonfat milk
- 1 tablespoon honey
- 2 large eggs
- 2 tablespoons canola oil
- 2 cups blueberries, divided
- 1/2 cup real maple syrup

Instructions

1 In a large bowl whisk together the flours, baking powder, baking soda and salt. In another bowl, beat together the buttermilk, non-fat milk, honey, eggs, and oil. Stir the wet ingredients into the dry ingredients, mixing only enough to combine them. Stir in 1 cup of berries.

2 Preheat a large nonstick griddle or skillet over a medium flame. Ladle the batter onto the skillet with a 1/4-cup measure. Flip the pancake when it is golden brown on the bottom and bubbles are forming on top, about 1 1/2 minutes. Cook the other side until golden brown, about 1 1/2 minutes. Serve topped with more blueberries and the maple syrup.

Nutrition Info

Calories: 324, Fat: 16g, Saturated Fat: 7g, Protein: 22g

☆☆☆☆☆

Rhubarb, Apple + Ginger Muffin Recipe

Prep/Cook Time: 50 mins, Servings: 8.

Ingredients

- 1/2 cup (55g) almond meal (ground almonds)
- 1/4 cup (50g) unrefined raw sugar
- 2 tablespoons finely chopped crystallised ginger
- 1 tablespoon ground linseed meal
- 1/2 cup (70g) buckwheat flour
- 1/4 cup (35g) fine brown rice flour
- 2 tablespoons organic cornflour or true arrowroot
- 2 teaspoons gluten-free baking powder
- 1/2 teaspoon ground cinnamon
- 1/2 teaspoon ground ginger
- a good pinch fine sea salt
- 1 cup finely sliced rhubarb
- 1 small apple, peeled, cored and finely diced
- 95ml (1/3 cup + 1 tablespoon) rice or almond milk
- 1/4 cup (60ml) olive oil
- 1 large free-range egg
- 1 teaspoon vanilla extract

Instructions

1   Preheat oven to 180C/350C. Grease or line eight 1/3 cup (80ml) cup capacity muffin tins with paper cases.

2   Place almond meal, sugar, ginger and linseed meal into a medium bowl. Sieve over flours, baking powder and spices,

then whisk to combine evenly. Stir in rhubarb and apple to coat in the flour mixture.

3   In another smaller bowl whisk milk, oil, egg and vanilla before pouring into the dry mixture and stirring until just combined.

4   Evenly divide batter between tins/paper cases (scatter with a few slices of rhubarb if desired) and bake for 20-25 minutes or until risen, golden around the edges and when a skewer is inserted into the centre it comes out clean.

5   Remove from the oven and set aside for 5 minutes before transferring to a wire rack to cool further.

6   Eat warm or at room temperature Best eaten on the day of baking, however they will store in an airtight container for 2-3 days or frozen in zip-lock bags for longer.

Nutrition Info

Calories 266, Protein 13 g, Carbohydrates 18g, Fat 5.4 g, Fibre 1 g

Crunchy Cinnamon Granola

Prep/Cook Time: 50 mins, Servings: 4

Ingredients

- 2 cups old-fashioned rolled oats
- 1/4 cup unsweetened shredded coconut
- 1/4 cup chopped walnuts
- 2 tablespoons pumpkin seeds
- 1/2 teaspoon ground cinnamon
- 1/4 teaspoon ground cloves
- 1/4 teaspoon ground nutmeg
- 1/4 cup honey

- 4 tablespoons unsalted butter, melted
- 1/4 cup raisins
- 1/4 cup chopped dried apricots
- 1/4 cup dried cranberries

Instructions

1 Preheat your oven to 300 degrees.
2 Line a baking sheet with parchment paper.
3 In a large mixing bowl, combine the oats, coconuts, walnuts, pumpkin seeds, and spices, and set aside.
4 Meanwhile, combine the honey and melted butter in a separate bowl, and pour it over the oat mixture. Stir well.
5 Spread the oat mixture out on the baking sheet. Bake for approximately 25 minutes, until golden. Remove from oven, and allow to cool.
6 Once cool, break up the granola, and mix in the dried fruit. Store in an airtight container.

Nutrition Info

Calories 190, Protein 14 g, Carbohydrates 20 g, Fat 5 g, Fibre 1 g, Sodium 638 mg.

Turmeric Rice Bowl With Garam Masala Root Vegetables & Chickpeas

Prep/Cook Time 50 m, 2 servings

Ingredients

Rice

- Vigo Authentic Spanish Recipe Saffron Yellow Rice 8 Oz

- 1 1/4 cups water
- 1/2 cup brown basmati rice
- 1/4 cup raisins
- 1 teaspoon extra-virgin olive oil
- Carapelli Firenze Organic Extra Virgin Olive Oil 17 Fl Oz
- 1 teaspoon onion powder or garlic powder
- 1/2 teaspoon ground turmeric or 1 teaspoon freshly grated turmeric
- 1/4 teaspoon ground cinnamon
- 1/4 teaspoon ground black pepper
- 1/8 teaspoon kosher salt

Vegetables & Chickpeas

- 2 tablespoons coconut oil or ghee
- 1 (15 ounce) can chickpeas, rinsed and patted dry
- 1 teaspoon garam masala or Indian curry powder
- 1 cup roasted root vegetables
- 1 teaspoon sugar or honey
- Domino Premium Pure Cane Granulated Sugar 4 Lb
- 1/4 teaspoon kosher salt
- 1/4 teaspoon ground pepper
- 2 tablespoons lemon juice
- 2 tablespoons low-fat plain yogurt or tahini
- Chopped fresh herbs, such as mint, parsley and/or cilantro, for garnish

Associated Recipes:

- Sheet-Pan Roasted Root Vegetables

Instructions

1   To prepare rice: Combine water, rice, raisins, olive oil, onion powder (or garlic powder), turmeric, cinnamon, pepper and 1/4 teaspoon salt in a small saucepan. Bring to a boil. Cover,

reduce heat to maintain a gentle simmer and cook until the li q uid is absorbed, 35 to 40 minutes. Remove from heat and let stand, covered, for 10 minutes. Meanwhile, to prepare vegetables & chickpeas: Heat coconut oil (or ghee) in a medium skillet over medium heat. Add chickpeas and cook, stirring, until crispy, 3 to 5 minutes. Stir in garam masala (or curry powder) and cook until fragrant, about 1 minute. Add roasted root vegetables, sugar (or honey), salt and pepper; cook, stirring often, until heated through, 2 to 4 minutes. Stir in lemon juice. Serve the vegetable mixture over the rice, topped with yogurt (or tahini). Garnish with herbs, if desired.

Nutrition info:

671 calories, 23 g fat, 14 g fiber, 107 g carbohydrates, 16 g protein; 175 mcg folate

Conclusion

A typical anti-inflammatory diet focuses on fighting inflammation through the consumption of foods that lower insulin levels. To actively reduce inflammation, you should therefore eat foods that have a low Glycemic load, such as whole grains, vegetables and lentils, and consume healthy fats such as nuts, seeds, fish, extra virgin olive oil and fish. Spices such as turmeric, ginger, and hot peppers also reduce inflammation. At the same time, you also need to reduce consumption of foods that are pro-inflammatory, such as red meat, egg yolks and shellfish. Sugar is a key culprit in inflammation, and therefore you should also cut back on sugary foods. Inflammation can also be reduced by taking supplements such as fish oils which are high in Omega 3 fatty acids.

www.ingramcontent.com/pod-product-compliance
Ingram Content Group UK Ltd.
Pitfield, Milton Keynes, MK11 3LW, UK
UKHW021709310125
4397UKWH00050B/565